Make YES an everyday affair.
Mardi Erdman

Mardi Erdman is co-owner and president of The Humanics Co.™, a Colorado-based firm offering programs on stress, fitness, and human resources. A stress management consultant and a certified yoga instructor, she has given classes and seminars all over the United States and in Europe.

Barbara K. Koplan is co-owner and vice president of The Humanics Co.™. She is a photographer, health and physical education intructor, and licensed paramedic and massage therapist.

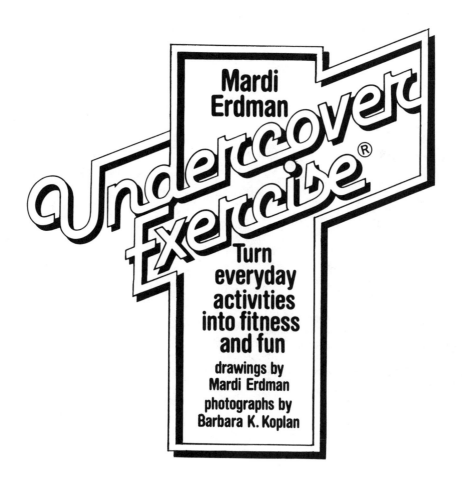

Mardi Erdman

Undercover exercise®

Turn everyday activities into fitness and fun

drawings by
Mardi Erdman
photographs by
Barbara K. Koplan

A SPECTRUM BOOK

Prentice-Hall, Inc., Englewood Cliffs, New Jersey 07632

Library of Congress Cataloging in Publication Data

Erdman, Mardi.
    Undercover exercise.

    "A Spectrum Book."
    Bibliography:
    Includes indexes.
    1. Exercise. 2. Yoga, Hatha. 3. Health. I. Title.
RA781.E73   1984   613.7'1   84-6772
ISBN 0-13-935453-0
ISBN 0-13-935446-8 (pbk.)

Editorial/production supervision: Inkwell
Page layout: Marie Alexander
Manufacturing buyer: Doreen Cavallo

This book is available at a special discount when ordered
in bulk quantities. Contact Prentice-Hall, Inc., General
Publishing Division, Special Sales, Englewood Cliffs, N.J. 07632.

A SPECTRUM BOOK

10 9 8 7 6 5 4 3 2 1

Printed in the United States of America

ISBN 0-13-935453-0

ISBN 0-13-935446-8 {PBK.}

Prentice-Hall International, Inc., *London*
Prentice-Hall of Australia Pty. Limited, *Sydney*
Prentice-Hall Canada Inc., *Toronto*
Prentice-Hall of India Private Limited, *New Delhi*
Prentice-Hall of Japan, Inc., *Tokyo*
Prentice-Hall of Southeast Asia Pte. Ltd., *Singapore*
Whitehall Books Limited, *Wellington, New Zealand*
Editora Prentice-Hall do Brasil Ltda., *Rio de Janeiro*

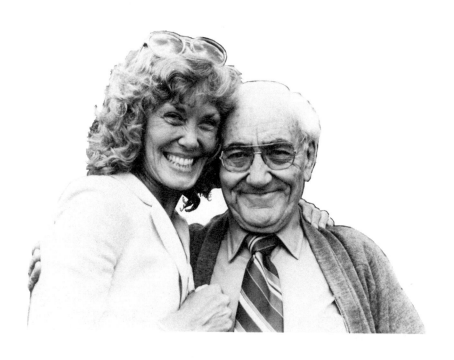

To Dad

and to the memory of Mother

Contents

3

Your Winning-Edge Workout:
Back and Body Trainers, 17

4

What Goes on Behind Bathroom Doors? 87

5

Undercover Antics on the Go, 94

6

Undercover Agents on the Job, 120

7

Under the Guise of the Mundane, 141

8

Under Your Covers, 162

9

Agents of Influence, 179

Forewords

A fundamental principal has been most beautifully restated through the recent discoveries of holographic physics. When applied to human experience, it says that the more a person is open, aware, connected to the infinite aspects of the universe, the more he or she is in touch with reality, and thereby whole.

In this time of superspecialization, rigid, narrow approaches to growth abound. Their names are countless, whether in therapy, religion, or philosophy. It is refreshing and important to find an approach that, although it stresses discipline, also stresses openness and attention to many aspects of daily existence in a most practical way. For many, *Undercover Exercise* will be a fun venture into a realm of everyday living that most of us have long neglected in our frequently misguided efforts to attend to "more important things." The results may well be a new zest for life in all its aspects.

Warren A. Baker, M.D.

It is the minority of our population that understands the interrelationship between the body and mind. Little interest is placed on the relationship of posture and wellness. Mardi, through personal experiences, has uncovered the reasons why so many of us in the western hemisphere suffer from a wide variety of ailments that are directly related to our sedentary lifestyle. Many cardiovascular diseases, musculo-skeletal disorders, and digestive abnormalities are related to our stressful existence and lack of understanding about the role of diet, posture, and exercise in wellness. The concepts, information, and energy derived from the practices explained in the pages of this book will allow one to reach the balance between mind and body essential for health and full living.

James R. Mosby, Jr., M.D.

Introduction

Here is a revolutionary way of living. It's simple. You can do UEs walking, standing in line, working at your desk or during anything you do. What are UEs? They are powerful exercises that ease backaches, headaches, relieve tension, and give you back your zest for life!

UEs are a way to get started in a new direction toward good health, good looks, and lots of laughs. They're so simple anyone can do them, yet they challenge you to do your very best.

This book teaches you to turn everyday life into a gold mine of workouts. You'll see pictures and read stories about people who are counteracting the deadly effects of sitting or standing in one place too long. You'll learn to use your chair as a health club and to work out as you shower, brush your teeth, travel, cook, shop, and even before you get out of bed.

Undercover Exercise

- increases circulation and gets a fresh blood supply to your brain,
- sharpens your wits,
- gives you a strong, supple spine, well oiled joints, beautiful skin, strong bones and muscles, free and natural breathing, and a way to get along better with people,
- boosts your spirits, teaches you how to bend, reach, and lift safely.

Undercover Exercise is a unique and simple way to weave a thread of undercover activity through your entire day. It's espionage—spying out ways to stretch and strengthen while you do all the things you usually do.

It all began when I was told I had osteoarthritis of the lower spine. Visions of myself confined to a wheelchair made me realize that I had to do something to help myself. In a very short time, I became totally immersed in a fascinating and absorbing game. I felt like Sherlock Holmes, scrutinizing my daily activities, analyzing my body in every standing, sitting, working, and playing position. What was hurting my back and what made it feel better? I was amazed (and amused) at how my thoughts and feelings affected my back tension.

Other authorities gave me helpful clues, but in the end, the work of applying the information was mine. I was already teaching and practicing yoga because yoga made me feel better, so I started experimenting with the yoga exercises while reaching for a dinner platter, bending over, or lifting. I found that I could do these exercises anywhere—at the store, in church, at the bank, or in meetings. They really made a difference! *They became my Undercover Exercise.*

As I studied and practiced I began to understand how my body was designed; and the relationship between my posture and my back problem. I learned that if I balanced my pelvis and elongated my spine, it took pressure off my lower back. This eased my back pain, and gave me a new way to stand and move.

There were others who needed the same kind of relief and help. I had despaired of ever teaching again when I first learned of my back problem. Instead of ending a career, it opened the door to an area of concern for millions of back sufferers. I began teaching these new concepts of body alignment, spinal extension, and stress management. I went to classes, workshops, seminars, studied books, and continued my own practice. The feedback from students and my television shows substantiated my own success with UEs. They worked! People were phoning and writing to tell me enthusiastically about how these exercises had changed their lives.

It was obvious that these principles of movement were helpful in many other ways. People with other kinds of problems felt better. Athletes moved better and had fewer injuries. People looked and felt better in their clothes and reported a new sense of well-being and self-confidence.

Undercover Exercise can turn *your* everyday actions into workouts. It's a love affair with life—a way of living ordinary life with extraordinary clarity and perception. This book will show you how to maintain vitality and youthfulness, relieve arthritic pain and stiffness, prevent the illnesses associated with stress, correct poor body alignment (posture), reduce medical costs, and alleviate "sititis" and "standitis."

In this book you will find:

- a Winning-Edge Workout for every day
- the essentials for a healthy body and a sound spine
- the Big Three Principles for using your spine safely
- a Be Sick-Get Better program
- a new way to get up in the morning
- a great way to go to sleep at night
- workouts for on the job
- UEs that make love lovelier
- ways to stay connected and whole in spite of the fragmentation of modern living

Read through Chapters 1 and 2. Do the Wake-Up Stretches in bed. You'll see that becoming an Undercover Agent isn't difficult, but you have to weigh the risks. If you decide to sign on, you'll discover the mystery and adventure of doing Undercover Exercise. It gives you a mission that's *not* impossible.

We salute each one of you who has inspired us—myself and Kope, the photographer—to record the courage, ingenuity, and humor in this book. Cheers to all you Undercover Agents—absorbed in a passionate love affair with life, giving it your full attention, doing the best that you can with the best that you have, to be the best that you are.

Acknowledgments

Here's to all of you who have made this book possible! Thank you to Advance Stationary, especially Steve Goldman; The Darkroom; Glenwood Springs Hot Pool and Athletic Club, especially Pat Rainey; Kally's Hardware, especially Wally Boals; Lakewood Camera; Monarch Printing; Montview Presbyterian Church, especially Reverend Ken Barley, Dr. Allen Maruyama, and Dr. Glendora Taylor; St. Paul's Community Church, especially Reverend Frank McCall; Robert C. Dorr; Richard Ebens; Stan and Pat Englehart; Dante and Meribeth Germanotta; Judy and Tom Kisselle; Cathe and Dick Kocak; A. Allen and Esther Koplan; Mary C. Lanius; Siegfried and Imgard Leistner; Gaye Lowe; Ron and Deena Prigosin; Rhodes Electric; Ditmar and Christa Schnittker; Arthur Stokes; Slater School, especially Dr. Mason; John Meininger; Norman B. Pester; Jan Sather; Bates and Robin Wilson, Lyn and Anne; Waxman Camera; Carol and Bob Whitney.

Thank you to Warren Baker, M.D., psychiatrist; Gerald S. Gordon, M.D., cardiologist and emergency medicine physician; Kaisel Steinhardt, M.D., orthopedic surgeon; and James R. Mosby, Jr., M.D., emergency medicine physician, for reviewing this manuscript.

Thank you to Prentice-Hall people John Kirk, Lynne Lumsden, Hal Siegel, and Fred Dahl for enthusiasm and expertise.

Thank you to my dear students, for all that they teach me; for their love, loyalty, and persistent search for excellence.

Thank you to my dear teachers for the light and wisdom they have given me, and especially to Mr. B.K.S. Iyengar, for teaching me the foundation of body alignment and yoga.

Thank you to Kope for steadfast perseverance, courage, integrity, humor, expert editing, and the splendidly fresh and spontaneous photographs that have made this project possible.

Thank you to Dad and Frances Bredemeier, Betty Earle, Don, Paul, and Julie Huffman for constancy and support.

Thank you to UEs for giving me the stamina and courage to move one step at a time.

Thank you to Jim, Chris, and Jamie for enduring the changes in our lifestyle, the transition in our roles, and for encouraging me to follow my dream.

Thank you to everyone who helps us follow our dreams.

1

Who Can Do Undercover Exercise?

*An idea becomes close to you only when you are
aware of it in your soul, when in reading about it it
seems to you that is has already occurred to you, that
you know it and are simply recalling it. . . .*
Tolstoy, *What Men Live By*

They are everywhere. Undercover Agents are operating in every nook and cranny of this planet. Highly trained and exquisitely aware, they are revolutionaries in the guise of ordinary people. They wear no uniforms, carry no cards, have no labels or insignias. If you watch carefully, you can spot them by what they do, how they do it, and the fruits of their actions. No other clues will reveal them, for they are young and old, rich and poor, of every color, race, and walk of life.

These Undercover Agents are involved in the most crucial espionage in history. Their work determines the survival of us all. Using different means and diverse schemes they are reclaiming this planet and proclaiming our birthright to be free and loving human beings.

It's all going on under our very noses. People everywhere, people you least expect, ordinary people like you and me are Undercover Agents (see Figure 1.1).

- They're looking life right in the eye! They are saying "I can and I will!"

- They're looking for excellence and a coherent lifestyle.
- They've got chutzpah and the confident belief that they make a difference.
- They've got the courage to endure and the stubborness to persist.
- They can use surprise tactics.
- They are keen observers.
- They are curious, concerned, and involved.
- They can empathize, pace, and be one with each other.
- They have finesse, tact, and polish.
- They know how to start, keep on, and persevere to the finish.
- They are negotiators, diplomats, strategists.
- They can spot a hoax and are nobody's fools.
- They take risks and learn from mistakes.
- They can extend themselves and stretch their minds, souls, and bodies.

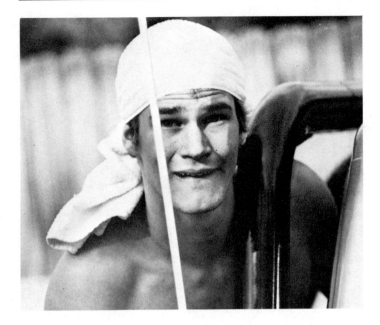

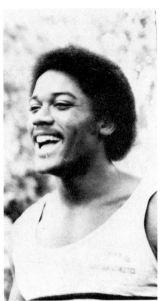

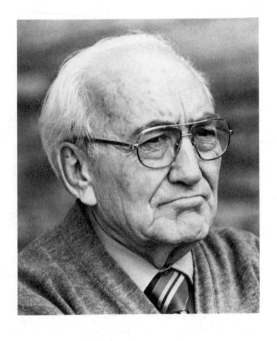

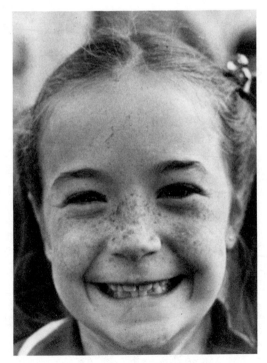

FIGURE 1.1

- They can laugh at themselves. They can cry. They know their belief systems and inner motivations.

- They refuse to be deluded by the easy answers or quick solutions to effects rather than causes.

Undercover Agents do *Undercover Exercise* to stay fit. *They are people doing the best that they can with the best that they have to be the best that they are.*

All of us do this to some degree unconsciously. Undercover Agents do it consciously, and the more conscious you are the less self-conscious you become. The less self-conscious you become, the better you can see, hear, touch, taste, smell, and sense the dynamics of life around you. *Undercover Exercise* affirms what we already know deep inside—what we are on the inside shows on the outside.

This book will teach you the essentials of good health and The Big Three Principles (Chapter 3) so that you can do whatever you want to do safely. You'll see other agents doing *Undercover Exercise* on the job, at home, anywhere. It's fun, intriguing, and easy to integrate into your own lifestyle.

First read this book, do the exercises, and learn the principles of proper breathing and movement. Then make it up as you go. Take what is appropriate for your mission . . . and go for it!

There are no membership fees and you don't need to buy a uniform. But you do need to assess the risks before you make your choice. If you decide to sign on, you need yourself and the full gamut of your resources. You will never run out of play or adventure that challenges your best. But remember, once you start there are no excuses. Undercover Agents can *always* find ways to do their Undercover Exercises! (See Figure 1.2.)

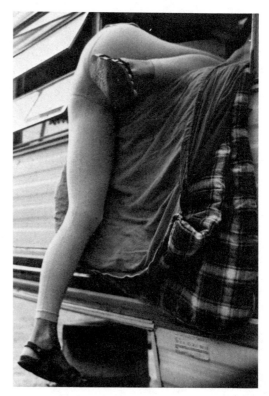

FIGURE 1.2

THE RISKS OF THE GAME

Everyday pressures collaborate with gravity to pull us down. Everydayism is a disease of stress and boredom that eats away at us like cancer. People frantically grope from one therapy to another for the "one true cure," a panacea for this disease. We secretly wish for the magic that would free the rigid minds and limbs that imprison us. For a while we try running, aerobic dance, meditation, chanting, yoga, Nautilus programs, or a new religion. Then the newness wears off and we realize that we're still stuck with ourselves.

The real risk is that we never get to what's eating us on the inside, that we live our whole lives without making peace with ourselves. We need heros—heros like you and me who will risk ourselves to find ourselves and help others to find themselves.

One of these heros is Kenneth Cooper, M.D., father of the aerobics revolution. In his latest book, *The Aerobics Program for Total Well Being*, he acknowledges that running is not the cure-all he dreamed it could be. He now emphasizes that running needs to be incorporated into a total lifestyle. I find that reassuring. I've learned that you can't be fit if you hate yourself and your neighbor. No matter how hard and long you run, the hate catches up with you. The running may discharge the feelings for a while, but it doesn't dissolve what's eating you!

In an interview, "John Naisbitts Monitors a Changing America," Naisbitts says that "the physical fitness trend . . . is not a fad . . . but an important and enduring change in lifestyles." (*The Tarrytown Letter,* Tarrytown, N.Y., April 1982, p. 10.) You know that! All you have to do is look at the ads, books, and magazines. They're full of it. And you've responded to the media blitz by joining health clubs, spas, buying new equipment, eating "wonder pills," and going on diets. And this is yet another book telling you how to get fit and stay healthy! Who needs it?

Ah . . . but wait. This book is about what you've known all along. Fitness begins with you. It's not in gimmicks and toys that entice for a while. Fitness progresses from the inside out. Who knows which comes first, fitness on the inside or fitness on the outside? Like the chicken and the egg, they are one; each needs the other.

Undercover Exercise brings the inside and the outside of us together. We get in touch with our inner selves. Something happens at the core of us, something quite like the Midas touch. Mundane actions are transformed into gold. Undercover Exercise takes common, ordinary work and turns it into an undercover workout . . . from the inside out! Emptying the garbage is like lifting weights, sweeping is like dancing.

What are the risks? There are risks in growing, but also in dying on the vine; in starting, but also in whether you can keep on and finish with style. There is risk in choosing your mission, your special part to play in this contemporary world; but greater risk in not having any sense of mission at all. Only you can decide what risks to take. And if you decide to risk Undercover Exercise, what are your pay-offs?

PAY-OFFS

Everybody loves a mystery. *Undercover Exercise* involves us in the mystery of who we really are, how we operate, and whether we can make the changes and choices for growth. It trains us in mastery of our minds through breathing and movement and rescues us from inertia and self-doubt. There is hope!

You can wish you were fit, wish you were fully alive, wish you had more energy, wish you were attractive, wish you could sleep at night, wish you didn't smoke, wish you didn't eat so much. But wishing doesn't cut it! It keeps you spreading out your backside while you eat French bonbons and watch TV. *Undercover Exercise* trains you to flip the mind-switch from "I can't" to "I can" and from "I won't" to "I will." It gives you that moment of personal power, personal choice. It gives you hope, for *hope is in the doing, not the wishing.*

It's tough out there. There aren't too many rose gardens! Every day we deal with monumental problems, some of us more than others. We all suffer through inflation, traffic jams, shoddy workmanship, and irresponsible and selfish people. We want to be appreciated and recognized by our associates but often get the feeling that no one cares. It's no wonder we suffer from stress and alienation.

Stress is a major cause of back pain. Four out of five Americans will suffer from back problems at some time in their lives; according to the latest figures, back problems put more of us out of commission than any other ailment except the common cold [1].

It stands to reason! The back is not just the spine but the head and the heart. What we think and experience is immediately transferred to our neck, shoulders, abdomen, hips, legs, and feet. We feel so fragmented and compartmentalized that we fail to realize the cause and effect of what we do. Hunched and scrunched shoulders send us home with a headache. Bending over to pick up a golf club can put our back into spasms and leave us bedridden.

Studying the Design Of Your Spine and The Big Three Principles in Chapter 3 doesn't necessarily mean that you'll have a trouble-free back. You have to implement what you learn by taking personal responsibility for your back and how you use it. Coming of age means becoming a Class A detective, finding out the cause and effect of things. You search for what has caused your headache, backache, or stomachache and zero in on treating the cause. You don't need to rely on tranquilizers or painkillers. Remember that a numb body is a dumb body. It can't tell you what is happening on the inside or outside because its sensitivity and intelligence have been deadened. You become a captive of the medication.

Class A detectives train daily both in The Winning-Edge Workout and throughout the day. The training sharpens your wits so that observing, checking, reevaluating, and discovering become a natural part of your skills. Like Sherlock Holmes, you may seem inordinately wise and uncanny to your peers; but in truth, you are just observant, sensitive, and aware. Yes, wise.

Merlin, the magician of King Arthur's court, was a genius of observation. Mary Stewart in her book *The Crystal Cave* makes a good case for what she believes is the magic of Merlin . . . *observation*. He observed everything, overlooked nothing, filed it all away in his computer brain. His magical powers were dramatic because no one else knew his secrets of observation. He could call up from his brain data to which no one else had access. He was magic! So are you! You too can train your computer brain in the keen power of observation. That's one of the big pay-offs of Undercover Exercise.

A side benefit of being a keen observer is that it dispels self-doubt and self-criticism. There simply isn't time for it. You are too busy noticing, gathering, collating, and storing information to be caught wallowing in self-pity. Not only is there no time for self-pity, but the "bad guys" miraculously start disappearing when you examine your own thoughts and actions. Self-examination is a big part of the detective work an agent encounters.

Learn from everything you do. Take risks and make mistakes. Mistakes are teachers. We go back and make it as right as we can, but the real profit is in learning from our mistakes. There is hope in learning.

Signing on requires three things:
1. *Spirit:* The spirit of curiosity and adventure, the ingenuity of our pioneering ancestors.
2. *Honor:* Honor yourself and that same inner self in others. Hold yourself in high esteem.
3. *Courage:* To do UEs to change your tack or to keep your course.

If you've decided to sign on, welcome aboard! If not, thank you for buying this book and please recycle it to a friend!

Undercover Agents, you are in league with other Agents who, in simple and grand ways, are on their mission. In disguise as housewives, doctors, teachers, bankers, secretaries, garbage collectors, students, carpenters, farmers, brick layers, and scores of other occupations, Undercover Agents are using the daily round to fulfill their mission. You have your own unique mission, so start immediately!

There are three basic rules of Operation Undercover Exercise:

1. Train in secret. Practice the New Way to Start Your Day and your Winning-Edge Workout. This secret training will give you the grace and strength for your mission. You can't execute your maneuvers in public without practicing them first in secret.
2. Start with vim, vigor, and vitality, but keep on with constancy, and finish with endurance.
3. Go undercover of it all. Seek out the core, your undercover core muscles (shown in Chapter 3, Figure 3.8). They are physical symbols of your inner source of power.

There are other pay-offs:

- You learn a whole new way to start your day, a way that will affect the rest of your day and everyone else's.
- Smokers can learn a way to kick the habit—taking a draw on your lungs instead of a cigarette. It does take consistent and persistent practice.
- Asthmatics and problem breathers can learn an easy UE that helps move the breath in and out of their lungs.
- Insomniacs can follow a ritual for sound and peaceful sleep.
- Families and partners learn to be together in new ways that promote communication, sharing, and loving.

You will discover other pay-offs as you practice UEs. Sign on as an Undercover Agent for the fun of it, the hilarity, health, strength, bounce and life of UEs. The pay-off is a body that works well for you and gets better every day. Older, but better! Are you ready to sign on now? Step this way, please.

SIGNING ON

Consider your options and then decide if you've got the heart for *Undercover Exercise.*

Don't sign on if you want any of the following:

1. To wallow in your misery.
2. To be scared of growing pains.
3. To be satisfied with doctor bills and bellyaches.

If that's not what you want, here is *your mandate:*

- Start with Chapter 2. Get yourself grounded and centered for the day.
- Review your mission and set your course.
- Train yourself in the Winning-Edge Workout in Chapter 3 so that you can do UEs throughout your day.
- Use strategic maneuvering, brilliant tactics, and the power of complete breathing in the bathroom, Chapter 4; on the go, Chapter 5; on the job, Chapter 6; in the mundane, Chapter 7; and under your covers, Chapter 8.

May the force be with you!

2

Undercover Take-Off: A New Way to Start Your Day

In the silence of deep night and in the quiet still
morning when the sun is touching the hills, there is
great mystery. It is there in all living things . . . In
the quiet stillness of the mind that which is
everlasting beauty comes, uninvited, unsought,
without the noise of recognition.
J. Krishnamurti, *Krishnamurti's Journal*

In the first fragile moments of the day you can go either way, toward your center or away from it. The alarm jangles at you, jarring your nerves, or the voice of the local DJ ushers in your morning with the same old Top 10. The news comes on with its plethora of heists, violence, and stock market reports. You can cover your head with your pillow and try for a few more minutes of sleep, but your peace has already been rudely shattered.

I used to wake every morning like that: I'd hear the news and weather, and then 15 minutes later roll out of bed as mentally preoccupied as if I'd been up for five hours!

Just as an experiment, I decided to try a different tack. I listened to myself for 15 minutes every morning . . . my real, very own inner voice. Goody, goody, I thought. I get to turn off the alarm and take 15 minutes to get in tune with myself and on top of my day. It made a difference! I found that if I heard the still, small voice in the early morning hours, it wasn't such a struggle to hear it later in the noise and din of my day.

Spiritual disciplines of every creed and religion have always stressed the need for early morning centering and alignment with the Ground of Being [2]. Tennyson said it so well: "If thou would'st hear the Nameless, and will dive into the Temple-cave of thine own self, there, brooding by the central altar, thou may'st haply learn the Nameless hath a voice, by which thou wilt abide, if thou be wise [3]."

We gave away the clock radio, and I got a little alarm that I could store under my pillow. Its muffled beep-beep didn't jar my predawn reverie. It alerted me to my time, my 15 minutes of being alone with myself. It has worked so well for me that I'm passing it on to you. I don't have to disturb my nice, warm husband, I don't have to get out of my nice, warm bed, and I can start the day in a nice, warm way.

Yes, it means changing routine. It means self-discipline and commitment. But there's just no way to skip discipline and still honor excellence.

You have to flip the mind-switch for this early morning start. It's the switch from "I can't" to "I can," "I won't" to "I will." No one can flip your switch for you. So here is your moment of personal truth. The time arrives. The beep-beep goes off. Are you or aren't you going to flip the switch? That moment has impact for you, your entire day, and everyone else around you. You have made a decision to choose your direction consciously. Time and time again throughout the day, that choice will come to you. What you do with your choices determines not only how you live your life but also, believe it or not, the state of the world!

BREATHING EXERCISES

Centering Alignment

- With the flip of the switch, turn over on your back and arrange yourself in alignment.
- Slide your hands under your buttocks and pull them outward and downward toward your feet. Then slide your hands out from under your hips.
- Press your back to the bed and flex your knees, elongating your spine. If you have back problems, keep a pillow ready to slide under your flexed knees.
- Then cross your arms over your chest and grasp your shoulders. Draw your shoulders down and away from your head.
- Release your hug and bring your arms beside your body, turning palms up.
- Gently roll your head from side to side until it centers. Your eyes are closed and you remain in a wonderful reverie state, half asleep, half awake. This ritual of paying attention to your body alignment is a very effective tool for mental and spiritual alignment.

Observer Breath

- Listen to your breath flowing in and out of you for several moments. Be attentive only to your breath. Like the lover with the loved one, you are fully aware, totally absorbed, and in complete oneness with your breath.
- Observe the innocence of the early morning breath. There is no trying, no striving . . . just breathing.
- Follow your breath as it passes in and out of your lungs for one minute (12-15 cycles). You'll find yourself untrained and undisciplined in the beginning. Your mind will wander and you may fall back to sleep. If that is a problem for you, get a snooze alarm that wakes you in five minutes. Then you can relax and not be anxious about oversleeping.
- Gradually increase the time that you are able to stay with your breath.
- Let the breath lead you into the temple-cave of your own self. Listen to the silence of your interior being.
- Observe how your brain can be conscious on many levels at once. One part of your brain can observe the other parts. This is sometimes referred to as the Observer Self.
- View the passing thoughts as if you were watching them parade across a TV screen.
- Watch. Develop the ability of keen observation without evaluating or judging. Like a court reporter, observe and note everything that is going on, but pass no judgment. Evaluating what you observe comes later, when making judgments is essential.
- Your passive breathing pattern is an early morning meditation, or mindfulness. All the breathing exercises that follow are active breathing patterns.
- Start with at least three cycles of passive

breathing to center and align yourself. The Observer Breath is one of your most powerful training and centering tools.

Abdominal Breathing

Although abdominal breathing is sometimes called diaphragmatic breathing, all breathing is actually initiated by the brain and diaphragm. In Abdominal Breathing, you are learning to use your abdominal muscles to assist your diaphragm. You will observe the relationship of lungs, ribs, the intercostal muscles between your ribs, diaphragm, and abdominal muscles. This kind of breathing lays the foundation for the Rhythmical Complete Breath. It helps you use your breath to power your own energy-generating plant.

Place your hands on your abdomen. Observe your breath moving in and out of your lungs and the subtle movement of your abdomen and ribs. Notice that as you breathe in, your abdomen moves out; as you breathe out, your abdomen moves in. Watch pets or babies while they sleep. They breathe the same way.

As the breath leaves your lungs, the diaphragm moves upward into the rib cage, assisting the emptying of the lungs, and your abdomen moves in. As the breath enters the lungs, the diaphragm moves downward and the abdomen moves out.

Many people try so hard in Abdominal Breathing that they overdo it. Don't make the mistake of forcing your breath or protruding your abdomen when you inhale. Just a little bit'll do ya! Concentrate on using the support of your contracting abdominal muscles as you exhale. You'll use this technique later in Rhythmical Complete Breathing. It'll help save your back from the stress and strain of daily living.

Now deepen your breath. As you inhale, relax and expand your abdomen without tensing it. Exhaling, draw your abdomen gently in toward your spine. Breathe in to a count of 3. Breathe out to a count of 6. Use a 1:2 ratio that's *comfortable* for you—2:4, 3:6, 4:8, or 5:10.

Use your nostrils as passageways, not pumps. They warm, humidify, and filter the air going into your lungs. Keep your throat full, as if stifling a yawn. This will give your breathing a full, deep sound, like Darth Vadar. But you should also be able to breathe very silently with your throat open, so that your breathing remains a secret resource undetectable to anyone but you.

In the beginning, do three cycles of breathing. Make your exhalations about twice as long as your inhalations. Breathe steadily and rhythmically. Eventually you'll be able to breathe like this for 5−10 minutes.

Whistle Breath

The Whistle Breath is for people who have difficulty exhaling or who have clogged nasal passages. Purse your lips and inhale as if you are sipping soda through a straw. Then whistle the breath out like air seeping out of a balloon. Try two or three cycles.

If deep or full breathing is difficult for you, take courage. Most people do not even begin to utilize this powerful and secret resource. Develop an awareness and appreciation for the breath that others take for granted.

If you have a bronchial condition or breathing problem, your doctor may have already recommended this Whistle, or pursed-lip breathing pattern. It calms you down and keeps you from panicking when you struggle to move your breath in or out of your lungs.

Now follow the procedure for Abdominal Breathing, but inhale through your nostrils and exhale through pursed lips. Do three cycles at first, exhaling about twice as long as you inhale. Remember that one cycle is one inhalation and one exhalation. Eventually you can increase the number of cycles.

Remember that you can't receive a full breath if you haven't gotten rid of the one you already have. Exhaling represents letting go, a surrender that can take us much farther than we can go on our own. This is a powerful, life-transforming meditation.

If you are a smoker who wants to quit smoking, this is a powerful ally. You *can* get hooked on fresh air instead of smoke! Do pursed-lip breathing on both inhalations and exhalations. Take a draw of air instead of a draw on a cigarette. Do three cycles at first, and then increase the number of cycles every time you want a cigarette. Don't overdo it! Focus on drawing in the life force, energy, instead of the cigarette smoke. It can work with the flip of your mind-switch from "I can't" to "I can" and "I won't" to "I will." It takes consistent and persistent practice. Calm yourself, and as you breathe, focus on what you really want. The breathing will give you time to look closely at yourself and zero in on what's really happening inside you.

Rhythmical Complete Breathing

Rhythmical Complete Breathing is a system of breathing that trains you to engage all the power and potential of your respiratory organs. As long as we live, we breathe. Most people breathe all their lives without knowing that they can be masters of their own power-generating plant, their breath. You can take this life force and generate power and light in your body, mind, and spirit.

Procedure

- Place one hand on your ribs and keep the other one on your abdomen.
- As you exhale, notice how your abdomen and ribs are drawn inward.
- As you inhale, feel the expansion begin low in your back and in the sides of your abdomen. Let it swell like the crest of a wave up through your chest, expanding the front, sides, and back of your rib cage.
- Pause for a moment at the top of your inhalation. This is the "hang time" of the breath, the silence equivalent to the in-

stant before a wave breaks into foam. This space holds the quiet of the inner self.

- Exhale slowly, feeling the wave of breath break and begin to recede again, lungs, ribs and abdomen returning to their empty state as the breath returns to its source. As you link your breath to the rhythm of the sea, experience in your own body the universal laws of expansion and contraction, ebb and flow, full and empty, work and rest.
- Inhale to a count of 3. Exhale to a count of 6. Make it a 1:2 ratio of inhalation (1) to exhalation (2). You may find that 4:8, 5:10, or 6:12 suits you better.
- Now try a rhythm of 1:1 ratio in which you inhale to a count of 3, 4, 5, or 6 and exhale to the same count. At the top of your inhalation and end of your exhalation, pause briefly and go into the "hang time" of your breath.
- *Stop if you feel dizzy or light-headed.* Breathe normally. Train yourself very gradually to do these fuller, deeper breathing patterns.

Spend your first waking moments in a state of relaxed awareness doing one or all three of the breathing exercises. Begin with the Observer Breath and go on to Abdominal Breathing. Once you are more awake, do Rhythmical Complete Breathing. With practice you can spend 5 to 15 minutes doing these breathing exercises.

It's best to do breathing exercises in clean, fresh air or filtered air. When we become aware of our breathing, we become aware of our planet and the air we all must breathe. There are fewer and fewer places where we can draw a fresh, clean breath of air. One of the best ways to clean up our air is to get people breathing again. Once you notice how dirty the air is, you're more willing to do something about it. Everywhere, Undercover Agents are fighting for their right to breathe.

By training your muscles to assist the lungs in filling and emptying, the lungs are better able to do their job of gas exchange. Your lungs will be stronger and better able to throw off the effects of pollution. Mr. B.K.S. Iyengar says in his classical treatise on pranayama, the art of breathing, that the breath is an energy, like a mighty river, that we can harness. If we master its power, we can provide vitality, vigor, and renewal for our systems. "Better breathing means a better and healthier life [4]."

MEDITATION

You may have already experienced meditation as you practiced Observer Breath, Abdominal Breathing, and Rhythmical Complete Breathing. You used the breath to link you with an inner reality that stabilizes, supports, and guides you.

Thomas Merton says in *New Seeds of Contemplation* that "contemplation is a sudden gift of awareness, an awakening to the Real within all that is real. A vivid awareness of infinite Being at the root of our own limited being. [5]"

You have probably read about all kinds of meditation. Is it chanting, counting beads, or repeating a mantra? Which method works? Systems and techniques are not meditation or contemplation; they are centering tools. They lead us gently but firmly beyond techniques and words to that which fills our souls with joy and love . . . the experience of the infinite at the core of our finiteness. We all have our belief systems and we have to find what satisfies our innermost souls. The methods we choose usually reflect the traditions in which we have been raised (Figure 2.1).

The following three focusing exercises calm your mind and help you meditate. Don't be trapped in mindless routine. It diminishes your awareness. If your mind won't settle down, shift to another breathing pattern or point of focus that completely engages you.

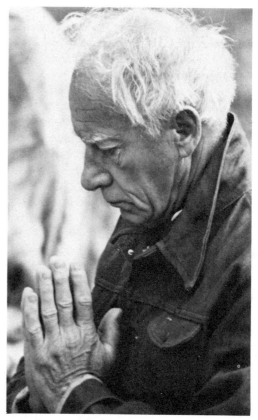

FIGURE 2.1

Counting Breaths

This ancient Zen meditation has always served to center me. I pass it on to you as a focusing meditation. Counting Breaths is a great technique for quieting mental fuming. Use it to keep your lid on when it's inappropriate to blow! Remember that old adage of counting to 10 before you vent your spleen? Well, it works. But some of us have to count to 20! It calms you and gives you a fresh perspective. Focus on your exhalations. Count them from 1 to 10 or 1 to 20 and back again from 10 to 1 or 20 to 1. Counting Breaths can anchor you to that feeling of centeredness. After a little practice, the first few counts can immediately calm you down and center you.

Humming Breath

This is such a simple but profound practice. As you exhale, hum like a bumblebee. Let the sound come from the depths of your being and reverberate through your body. Hum whatever tone feels good to you; don't worry about sounding wonderful yet!

Are you humming in your throat? If so, your hum will be weak and ineffectual. Let the sound arise from the depths of your abdomen and pass through your throat into your head. Don't be timid about it. Let it buzz with energy and vibration behind your eyes, forehead, nose, and lips.

This exercise develops voice volume and projection ability. It has changed weak, whiny singers and speakers into dynamic, powerful ones. Lawyers, salespeople, singers, teachers, politicians, and clergy have used this Humming Breath to change their self-concept and projected image. You can too!

Practice the Humming Breath while you're driving. This is for solo trips! Imagine that you can pierce the windshield with a laserlike beam of sound vibrations! It can get you ready for your next appointment in high style! And not only that, humming is great entertainment while you drive. Put an *M* or *N* in front of vowels, making "Ma Mu Ma Mu" and "Na Nu Na Nu." Try it; it's fun!

Humming, whistling, or singing while you work is a great way to reduce stress. Remember that lyrics have a powerful effect on you, so carefully choose your song. It's so easy to take on someone else's sad love affair! But the greatest classics, folk songs, and spirituals inspire our hearts and wills.

The Gift of Life Meditation

Every day is a gift, a gift of life and opportunity. This is a powerful meditation for celebrating life. *L'chaim!*

Focus on your breath flowing in. It's the gift of love and life. The alchemy of your body transforms and uses it. Then you give it back as the breath flows out again. Other forms of life will use it and send it back to you.

The gift of breath is a continual reminder of how we are all linked together, how we give and receive in the miracle of life. The gift of breath helps us understand and experience the gift of love. Like breath, loves comes into us and arises from our depths. We don't fully understand it but receive it as a gift. It makes little miracles happen inside and then flows out to others. It nourishes and sustains us all. Love is the most powerful healer we know.

The breathing and focusing exercises you have just learned can be done either lying in bed, sitting, standing, or walking. Sit in Tailor Pose (ankles crossed) or Bound Angle (Chapter 3). You can lean against the wall or headboard for support, but keep your back straight.

Meditation has active and passive phases. It can be a quiet time of sitting or an active workout, as described in the following chapter.

Most of us need the discipline of a time and place designated for meditation. It can be first thing in the morning when you practice your breathing and centering exercises or you can set aside a time for sitting or walking meditation (Figure 2.2).

Begin with one of the focusing exercises: Counting Breaths, Humming Breath, Gift of Life Meditation, or start your sitting meditation with a short reading from a devotional book or scriptures of your faith. Reflect for a moment on what the passage means to you. Use a phrase from what you've read, a thought, verse, or poem, as a point of focus. Repeat it rhythmically as you breathe. This is helpful when your mind is doing gymnastics and you want to settle down.

Here are some phrases that mean a lot to me:

- Be still my soul, all is well.
- I have what I need.

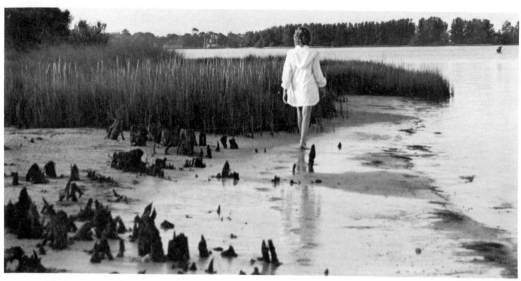

FIGURE 2.2

- "Thou art my strength and my shield; of whom shall I be afraid?"

The important thing is that these exercises lead you into a period of quiet where you can go beyond the words and ideas. If you are always holding a dialogue with yourself or convincing yourself that everything is all right, how can you ever get to what's eating you inside? We must see ourselves clearly and wrestle with the deeper issues of our motivations if we want to get to the heart of our lives.

Sometimes seeing is very disturbing. Whatever your spiritual discipline, this quiet time is not always peaceful. There seems to be no peace of mind and there are no easy answers. German theologians call this *Die Unruhe des Glaubens*, the restlessness of faith. If you are experiencing this at least you know you've gotten beyond the mask each of us tries to hide behind. It is painful. But in the restlessness of doubt, there is the faith that we can find ourselves, our real selves.

This kind of confrontation brings the peace of aligning ourselves again and again with what the theologian Paul Tillich calls "Ground of Being [6]." That's why the UEs are so powerful: they are physical, mental, and spiritual exercises that align our bodies and center our minds.

WAKE-UP STRETCHES

The birds do it, the bees do it, your pets do it. Why don't we do it? I was watching a sparrow this morning. His Two-Way Stretch was phenomenal! He pushed his little feet down on the roof of the rabbit hutch and his whole body, from legs to beak, elongated. Have you ever noticed how often animals stretch?

These five Wake-Up Stretches in bed will help you to stretch and elongate your body. Before your feet even hit the deck, you'll feel alive and ready for your day. The rhythmical breathing, with slow, coordinated movements, will give you an added bonus. It'll get your body's immune system going and bring a rich, nurturing blood supply to every cell in your body.

Here you go undercover!

Alignment Stretch

- Lying on your back, quietly fold your arms over your chest and grasp elbows.
- Take your arms over your head as you inhale.
- Exhale and stretch your elbows toward the wall behind you. Stretch. See if you can keep your arms on the bed.
- Inhaling, point your toes and gently arch your chest.
- Exhaling, flex your feet and flatten your back to the bed.
- Do these movements for 12 to 15 cycles of breathing.
- Relax and feel the life force tingling through your veins.
- Wiggle and squiggle your whole body into the bed like a bowl full of jelly.

The next four exercises are described more completely in Chapter 3.

Knee-to-Chest Squeeze

- Bend one knee and grasp the back of your thigh. Remain undercover!
- Exhaling, squeeze your knee to your chest. Keep the opposite leg stretched along the bed or bent, with your foot resting on the bed.
- Inhaling, release the squeeze and let your ribs expand with the breath.
- Do five squeezes and then switch legs and do five more.

Huggy Pose or Turkey Pose

- Bring both knees to your chest and grasp the backs of your thighs.
- Exhaling, squeeze your knees to your chest.
- Inhaling, release the squeeze and expand your chest.
- Continue the squeeze-release a few more times.

- Add the Head Roll-Up on your exhalations, bringing your forehead toward your knees.
- Vary Huggy Pose with the Turkey Pose by spreading your legs wide apart. Continue squeezing your thighs to your sides as you exhale, releasing the squeeze as you inhale. Keep your head relaxed on the bed throughout Turkey Pose.
- Do these rhythmical squeeze-release movements for 12 to 15 breathing cycles, or for about one minute.
- For icing on the cake, hold the squeeze in either Huggy or Turkey pose for three to five minutes. Great for bad backs and pains in the neck! You can also do this before going to sleep at night.

Easy Back Twist

- Slide one leg out on the bed in alignment with your hip joint, keeping the other knee bent.
- Grasp the bent knee with the opposite hand.
- Exhaling, draw the bent knee across your body toward the opposite side as far as you can or until your knee touches the bed.
- Let the opposite arm hang loosely at your side.
- Turn your head in the opposite direction of the bent knee.
- Keep your free arm and both shoulders on the bed throughout the pose.
- Exhaling, roll back to center and quietly do the pose with the opposite leg bent.

Cobra Pose

- Roll over and slide a pillow under your abdomen.
- Stretch your arms out in front of you until they touch the headboard or wall.
- Inhaling, expand your ribs.

- Exhaling, draw your abdomen inward, toward your spine.
- Tuck your pelvis. See Chapter 3, Back Trainers, for further assistance.
- Walk your hands 6 to 12 inches up the wall or headboard. You can also just keep your hands on the bed in front of you.
- Use the wall or bed to push against as you lift your head and chest off the bed. Breathe rhythmically, expanding your ribs on inhalations. Draw your abdominals firmly toward your spine on exhalations.
- Notice what pushing against the wall does for you. Any resistance you may encounter today can be just like this wall; it can lift you and make you stronger.
- Release the stretch and rest on your bed. Repeat the pose again if you wish. It stimulates the energy in your spinal column and helps you wake up all over.
- Curl up on your left side in a fetal position and breathe quietly for a few moments.

Relax, be still, and let go of tension in your muscles. Imagine space between your joints. Be aware of all the sensations feeding into your brain. This is a time when ideas often take form. Many good solutions to perplexing problems occur in this quiet time. Occasionally you may want to jot down thoughts that come to you. If a poem, verse, aphorism, or song comes to mind, take it with you throughout the day. Utilize what you hear from within.

Take a moment either in this curled-up pose or sitting or walking meditation to plan your day and set your course. Then let go. You've prepared for what the vagaries of life will bring you. Review your purpose and mission in life. Turn it into a statement or aphorism that reveals what you feel is your reason to be alive. Then check your plans for

congruence with your mission. This helps you to know when to change tack or keep your course.

Nietzsche said, "He who has a *why* to live can bear with almost any *how*." Focus your attention on the process of your day, not the product. Like the sand sculptor (Figure 2.3) focus on the doing. He knows that the tide will wash away his work of art but it can't take his love, concentration, and joy of creation.

I am always amazed at the effect the Breathing Exercises and Wake-Up Stretches have on me. Others say the same. It seems that these 10 to 15 minutes have more impact than 30 to 60 minutes of the same routine later in the day. Perhaps it's due to the open, receptive, vulnerable state of body-mind early in the morning. Or perhaps it's the psychological edge you give yourself when you flip the mind-switch from "I won't" to "I will." Whatever the reason, the effect is phenomenal! You can roll out of bed knowing that you have touched base with your internal and external resources and that with them, you can handle anything that comes along this day.

TIPS FOR A NEW DAY

- As you awaken, become mindful of that presence within you that neither slumbers nor sleeps. Be grateful for a new day and the chance to live it.
- When the alarm goes off, you don't have to get out of bed. Flip the mind-switch and breathe the stuff of life for a powerful start.
- Review your day and make your plans with alternatives for contingencies. Count on everything going wrong that can go wrong! Cartoon it!
- Check your plans and goals with your mission, the fundamental purpose and meaning of your life. Have you set your sail in the direction of your course?
- Be careful not to become rigid. Goals

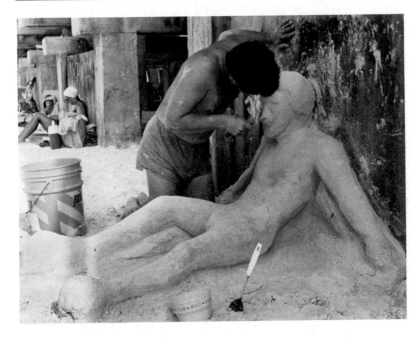

FIGURE 2.3

create tension if everything has to go according to a master plan—yours or anyone else's.

- Look at your dreads. Face them squarely and see what you can learn from them. Dreading is worse than the dread itself.
- Think of someone you'll meet today who really makes you smile, like the cheerful face in Figure 2.4. Your day seems better already.
- Remind yourself that you have new resources. UEs give you new ways to exorcise old problems.
- Look forward to your Winning-Edge Workout where you can practice your UEs. Remember, *you can't be in public what you haven't practiced in private.*

Think of the most difficult person you will encounter today. Send that person a "Love Missile." Pretend he or she is surrounded with enough love to overflow inside. Eyes shine and that face is content and

happy. Visualize the very best this person could want to happen. This is a very difficult exercise—the hardest in this book—but the results are astonishing! Try it and see. The profit is worth the effort.

Now up and at em! Go on to your Winning-Edge Workout, Chapter 3, or carry on in the bathroom, Chapter 4.

FIGURE 2.4

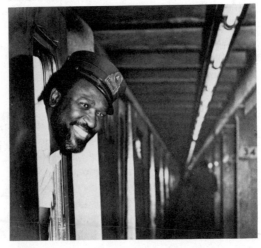

3

Your Winning-Edge Workout: Back and Body Trainers

The choice today is not between escape and disaster. It
is, as it always was, between the satisfactions that blind
and the obligations that awaken.
Norman Cousins, *Human Options*

If you think you have lost your suppleness
and spontaneity, the Back and Body Trainers
will help you get them back. If you've got
them, these UEs help you keep them. They
are the framework of Undercover Exercise.

As a child you did these things as a
natural part of your play. Your body remembers them. The exercises may be a struggle at
first because of stiffness and your own resistance to change. Invest a little time and soon
you'll feel as if you've come home again to a
very natural but long forgotten part of you.

The winning edge that puts you across is
everyday practice like any artist or athlete.
Your workout becomes a "positive addiction," as William Glaser calls it in his book by
that title. You have to have it! You feel subhuman without it. Learn just one configuration like One-Leggers and you will find yourself transforming common everyday activities
into valuable workouts. Brushing your teeth
becomes the workout you've got time for
right now (see Figure 3.1). Hanging from the
handrail of the subway train on the way to
work turns transit time into training time.

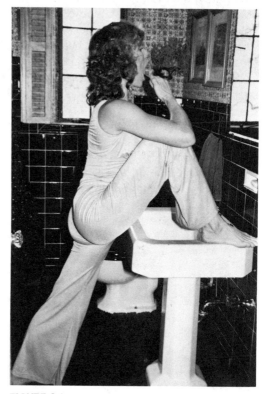

FIGURE 3.1

Your dividends depend upon what you put into the training bank. What you put in you get back a hundred-fold! Watch it happen. You'll love it.

Your Winning-Edge Workout has two parts: Back Trainers and Body Trainers. Back Trainers teach you about your spine and how to keep it strong, stable, and supple. They help you with back problems, including recuperation from injury or surgery. Body Trainers build on the foundation of Back Trainers. They develop strength, endurance, and good body alignment. Your Aerobic Workout, as part of Body Trainers, expands your Undercover Exercise to include the fun and de-stressing of aerobic activities.

WHAT'S YOUR HISTORY?

You were a baby once. Look at Figure 3.2A; your spine looked like that. You couldn't do anything for yourself except suck and cry. Then you learned to lift your head, grasp, focus your eyes and crawl. Your spine began to form curves that would be vital to your strength and flexibility. (See Figures 3.2B and C.)

As you began to use your body for new tasks, your environment and genetic inheritance determined the ways in which you moved. These patterns became habitual, and before long your body began to reflect your very own way of moving in the world. One side of you probably became dominant—

shorter or longer or more massive or higher than the other. The older you got, the less freely your body seemed to move. You got accustomed to the misalignment, the unevenness. Soon the joints began to forget their full range of movement, and your movements were tighter and more restricted. You were grown up before you knew it. And being an adult seemed synonymous with stiffness and a spare tire around your waistline.

But the early freedom of movement has never left your memory. You get glimpses of it now and then watching a superb athlete or a child. Within you stirs the longing to move that way again.

What does it take to get that youthful freedom of movement back? You may be weary and leary of the new-age gimmicks aimed at self-improvement. Undercover Exercise gives you a way to be strong and flexible doing what you do every day anyway! Look at the photographs throughout this book of people like you doing everyday things. Look at the possibilities of working out wherever you are. You don't need anything new or gimmicky. All you need is what you've got!

WHAT CAN YOU DO WITH WHAT YOU'VE GOT?

What you've got is all your equipment. Your brain and spinal column are the core for all movement. Learning to take care of your spi-

FIGURE 3.2

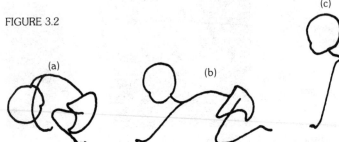
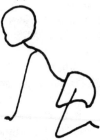

(a)   (b)   (c)

nal column is a 24-hour vigil. It's a secret watch for things that harm your back and for ways to make your spine *strong, stable,* and *supple.*

Some of you were born with a normal spine, others were not. Some of you, because of life's circumstances, find yourself with difficult challenges. I've taught classes in which there were people blind, deaf, partially paralyzed, in body casts, and with back problems. We all left class each week aware of our limitations but very glad for what we had!

Each of you is unique. You have to do the best with what you have! And some of you will far outdo the rest in grit and determination. Adapt, improvise! Be flexible about what you can do with whatever you've got. Time and again you'll see photographs in this book of people who've learned to apply that principle.

THE ORIGIN OF BACK AND BODY TRAINERS

Back and Body Trainers are the heart of any good and continuing program for a healthy spine. They come from years of experience teaching myself and others how to combat back pain, poor posture, and stressful thoughts. They come from programs of physical therapists, suggestions of orthopedic specialists, and the ancient art of yoga.

Why yoga? Because yoga, practiced artfully and precisely, contains the essential ingredients for a healthy back and body: *circulation, alignment,* and *extension.*

In 1976 my back pain took me to the specialists. One of my doctors prescribed a back brace and aspirin for my back pain. My good sense told me I'd learn nothing, grow weaker, and have to rely on the back brace and aspirin forever. Yoga increased my circulation (goodbye, aspirin), aligned my spine (goodbye, back brace), and taught me to extend my spine and limbs. It gave me faith in myself.

That doesn't mean that you need to throw away the back brace and aspirin. They can give you the support and relief you need while you *learn* the Back Trainers and *understand the cause* of your problem. Get your physician's approval before you begin.

The Back and Body Trainers are based on ancient yoga asanas that are designed for spinal health. Whenever possible, I use the Sanskrit name for classification and reference purposes. *Asana* means posture or pose. It is a place to be for a while, to find out what parts of you are out of balance, where your energy is going, and how your thoughts affect your body. They teach you the art of focus and concentration . . . the mother of all the arts.

With daily practice, you will naturally begin to assume proper sitting, standing, sleeping, and working postures. You will know when you are standing with one hip stuck out, driving with your head and chin thrust forward, or straining your back while lifting. As one student put it, "Your everyday habits begin to feel yukky! Then you really have to either resign yourself to feeling yukky or change it."

The yoga system of rhythmical breathing and moving is the perfect foundation for your Undercover Exercise. First, you will increase circulation to *every* part of your body. It's probably starving in places, suffocating in others! Blood is your lifeline. Blood, with the oxygen and nutrients it carries to your cells and the waste products it carries out of your cells, heals you and keeps you healthy. This is essential to life itself.

Second, yoga's centering and precision alignment of your whole body help you correct old habits that cause wear and tear on joints and ligaments. You wouldn't dream of driving on new tires without an alignment job. Yoga is like an alignment job on your body.

Third, you will use the force of gravity to help lift and elongate your spine, creating extension. You'll look taller, poised and confident.

BACK TRAINERS

Back Trainers are designed to reeducate your spine, your core. Master these asanas (poses) first, and they will give you freedom in moving and breathing. They work out tension so you will be able to relax. They are what they say they are . . . back trainers. They give you back your back—strong, stable, and supple. They work!

When you understand the simple principles of movement in Tip and Tuck, Cosmic Sandwich, and Dynamic Duo, you will be able to apply your knowledge of healthy back principles to the Body Trainers and everything else you do.

Consult your doctor, physical therapist, or trainer (priest, rabbi, or mother). Decide which exercises are best for you to do. Start with these daily, and don't be surprised if you feel a little sore or achy at first. Your muscles and joints need gentle but persistent training. Don't overdo and become overtired. That could discourage you. But *do* challenge yourself safely. If you don't feel your muscles, you know you haven't given them anything fun and interesting to do lately.

Most important, think, and feel these exercises as completely as you can. Breathe with them. Go under the cover of what you do, go into it. Imagine that you can see your skeleton moving—the joints of your spine moving, your hinge joints opening and closing, your ball and socket joints well oiled and rotating smoothly. Feel the muscles that are contracting and relaxing. Just a few minutes of this focus and attention is rejuvenating. You'll be amazed at the universe within you. And the more you notice, the more there is to notice. The fascination is endless.

The Design Of Your Spine

Now take a look at the core, your spine (Figure 3.3). Do you see how well designed it is? Its S-shaped primary and secondary curves

FIGURE 3.3

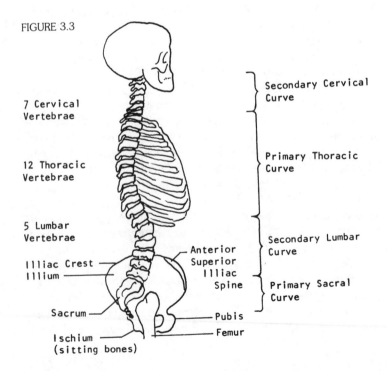

7 Cervical
Vertebrae

12 Thoracic
Vertebrae

5 Lumbar
Vertebrae

Illiac Crest
Illium

Sacrum

Ischium
(sitting bones)

Anterior
Superior
Illiac
Spine

Pubis

Femur

Secondary Cervical
Curve

Primary Thoracic
Curve

Secondary Lumbar
Curve

Primary Sacral
Curve

make it a very stable and strong backbone.

The bones of the spine are called *vertebrae*. There are four kinds: 7 *cervical*, 12 *thoracic*, 5 *lumbar*, and 5 *sacral*. The tailbone, or *coccyx*, is the last of the sacral vertebrae. The vertebrae are threaded together like pearls on a string to protect the spinal cord and nerves, and to provide movement of the torso.

You were born with two *primary curves:* thoracic and sacral. The first of the *secondary curves*, the cervical, developed as you began to lift your head. (Look again at Figure 3.2, A and B.) The next secondary curve, the *lumbar*, developed as you learned to balance the body in an upright position (Figure 3.2C). These secondary and primary curves of your spine give it strength and stability, as well as flexibility.

A perfectly straight spine would severely limit strength and flexibility. A spine with exaggerated secondary curves is weak and has difficulty accommodating stress. But the normal human spine with primary and secondary curves that evenly distribute stress throughout the column, is *strong, stable,* and *supple*.

Let's look at your skeleton (Figure 3.4, A and B). Notice that there are two potentially weak places where the spine is not supported by other bones. They are the cervical and lumbar spine. You know from experience that the neck and lower back are areas of stress, strain, and pain.

The head has to be supported by the cervical spine, and that is a little like trying to balance a watermelon on a bamboo fishing pole. Look at how the seven cervical vertebrae curve to the anterior, or front, of the body. The vertebrae are supported by muscles, tendons, and ligaments. If the head is carried too far forward, the cervical curve is too straight. If the head is carried too far back, the curve is exaggerated. Either condition will eventually lead to deformity, back pain, and headache. So much can be done to help prevent and

correct this "turkey neck" condition. (See Figure 3.5.)

The lumbar vertebrae are the weight-bearing vertebrae of the body. Look at the job those five lumbar vertebrae have to do all by themselves. The sacral spine is fused and gets support from the pelvis. The thoracic spine is supported by the ribs. But the valiant lumbar vertebrae do their job without any support from other bony structures.

In order for these vertebrae to maintain the proper curves of the spine, they must have support from the muscles, tendons, and ligaments of the abdomen and back. When the curve of the lumbar vertebrae is too exaggerated, the structure is weak and forms a curve called lordosis or swayback (Figure 3.6).

In swayback, the abdominal muscles in the front of the body are not adequately supporting the spine and balancing the pelvis. The back muscles are actually being over-stressed. They are shortened and contracted to compensate for the lack of abdominal support. Because the spine is out of alignment, the posterior (toward the back) sides of the lumbar vertebrae can be jammed together, causing the discs between the vertebrae to compress (see Figure 3.7). Dr. Paul Williams refers to the discs as jelly donuts and the vertebrae as hockey pucks. [7] If the spaces between the vertabrae are not maintained, the jelly donuts get squooshed. Out comes the jelly! The gelatinous substance inside ruptures the outer wall of the disc and presses against the nerves. This is called a ruptured disc. If the outer wall of the disc bulges, the condition is called a slipped disc.

What keeps the discs from getting squooshed between the vertebrae in the lumbar and cervical spine? The balanced training of muscles above and below, in front and in back of the spinal column keeps your vertebrae aligned and properly spaced one on top of the other. That's what the Big Three Principles are all about.

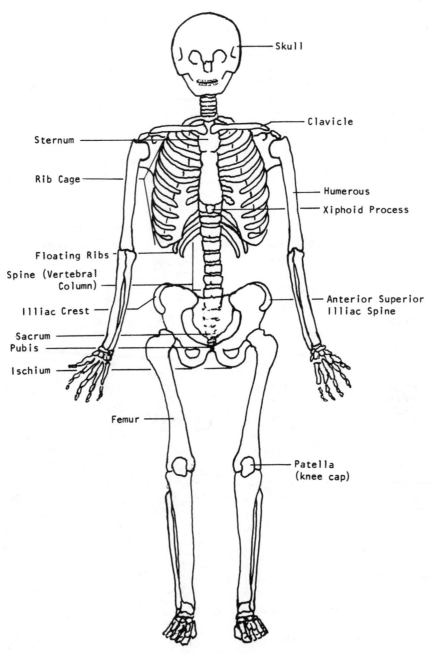

Skull

Clavicle

Sternum

Rib Cage

Humerous

Xiphoid Process

Floating Ribs

Spine (Vertebral Column)

Illiac Crest

Anterior Superior Illiac Spine

Sacrum
Pubis

Ischium

Femur

Patella (knee cap)

FIGURE 3.4(a)

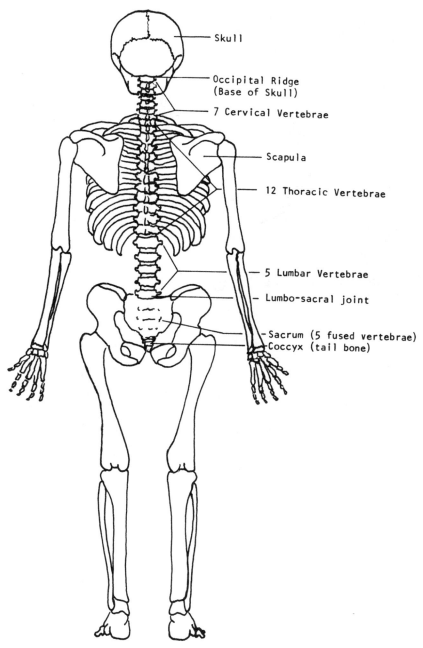

Skull

Occipital Ridge
(Base of Skull)

7 Cervical Vertebrae

Scapula

12 Thoracic Vertebrae

5 Lumbar Vertebrae

Lumbo-sacral joint

Sacrum (5 fused vertebrae)
Coccyx (tail bone)

FIGURE 3.4(b)

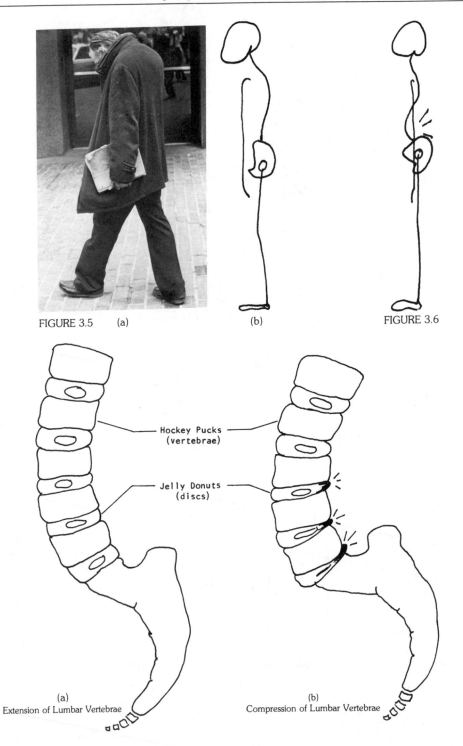

FIGURE 3.5   (a)   (b)   FIGURE 3.6

Hockey Pucks
(vertebrae)

Jelly Donuts
(discs)

(a)   (b)
Extension of Lumbar Vertebrae   Compression of Lumbar Vertebrae

FIGURE 3.7

Study the muscles of the body, both the superficial muscles (Figure 3.8, A and B) and the cutaways of the undercover muscles (Figure 3.8C and D). Refer to them frequently as you learn these dynamic principles of how to move your body.

The Big Three Principles

Here they are! The Big Three Principles in Back Trainers are Tip and Tuck, Cosmic Sandwich, and Dynamic Duo. They will train you to keep your spine strong, stable, and supple.

Tip and Tuck   Tip and Tuck will teach you how to rotate your pelvis so that your spine moves rhythmically with your pelvis, enabling you to bend and move with the least strain to your lumbar vertebrae and discs. You will learn this principle as you practice Supine Tip and Tuck, Table Pose, Cat-Cow, and the Fulcrum-Lever Concept in bending, lifting, and reaching.

Wherever you are, lie down on the floor or ground. Bend your knees and place your feet on the floor. Let your arms lie loosely at your sides. Take a moment to visualize your spine with its primary and secondary curves.

Feel the curve of your skull resting on the floor. Now with one hand, see how much space there is between the floor and your neck. This is the secondary curve of your cervical spine—from base of skull to shoulders. See if you can press the back of your neck to your hand. If you can't, you need practice in lengthening the muscles at the back of the neck.

Another way to check your cervical curve is to see if your chin is perpendicular to the floor. If it tilts backward, you need to place a folded towel, blanket, or firm pillow under your head while doing any exercises on your back (supine). Make the pillow just high enough so that your chin is perpendicular to the floor and your throat relaxed.

Follow your thoracic curve through the middle of your back. This is one of your primary curves. If you have a pronounced thoracic curve, you probably have rounded shoulders and/or a turkey neck. If you have massive shoulders and back muscles, as some weight lifters do, your head will drop too far backward. Use a cushion under your head.

Trace your spine as it curves inward again. This is your other very vulnerable secondary curve. Place your hand underneath the lumbar. See how much room you have between the floor and your lower back. If you do have a lot of space there, you are either arching your back or you may have swayback.

See if you can press your back firmly to your hand or the floor. That's the tuck. The tuck is very important to people with swayback, especially when they stand, walk, or run. Notice your thighs, buttocks, and abdominal muscles working together. Just hold that for a minute and visualize spaces being created between your vertebrae, relieving compression.

Now let your legs slide out, and lie on the floor with your legs extended. That usually increases your lumbar curve. Flatten your back to the floor again. It will be harder to do now than in the flexed- (bent-) knee position. This will help you to understand what you have to do while standing, since standing is also an extended-leg position. If you have trouble pressing your back to the floor, flex your knees slightly. Notice how much you have to bend your knees to lengthen the lumbar curve.

Here comes the last curve, the sacral. Feel the bony structures of the sacrum, which feels like a saucer. In the Tuck position, notice how the back rim of your pelvis and your sacrum press into the floor. Your buttocks may also lift slightly, but your waistline stays down when you practice the Tuck.

Supine Tip and Tuck.   Now you know a little more about your spine. Clasp your hands be-

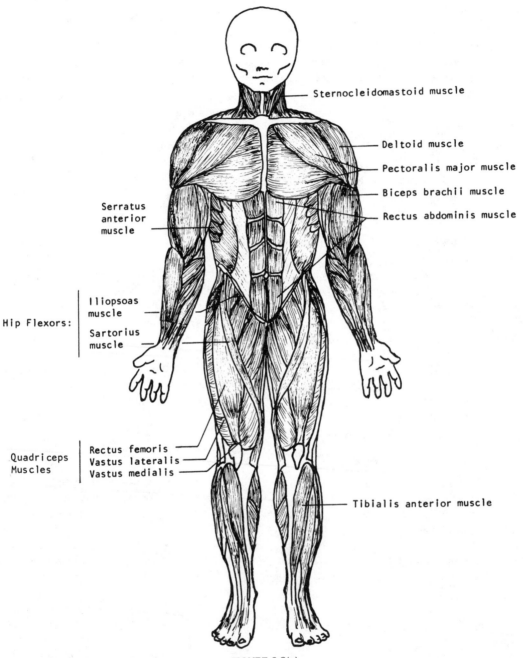

Sternocleidomastoid muscle

Deltoid muscle

Pectoralis major muscle

Biceps brachii muscle

Rectus abdominis muscle

Serratus
anterior
muscle

Hip Flexors: Iliopsoas
muscle

Sartorius
muscle

Quadriceps
Muscles

Rectus femoris
Vastus lateralis
Vastus medialis

Tibialis anterior muscle

FIGURE 3.8(a)

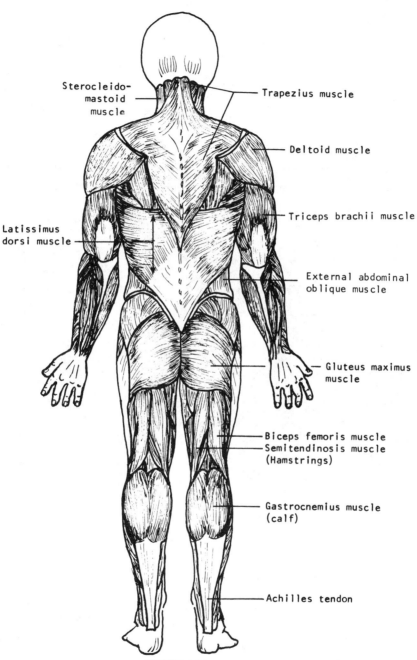

Sterocleido-
mastoid
muscle

Trapezius muscle

Deltoid muscle

Triceps brachii muscle

Latissimus
dorsi muscle

External abdominal
oblique muscle

Gluteus maximus
muscle

Biceps femoris muscle
Semitendinosis muscle
(Hamstrings)

Gastrocnemius muscle
(calf)

Achilles tendon

FIGURE 3.8(b)

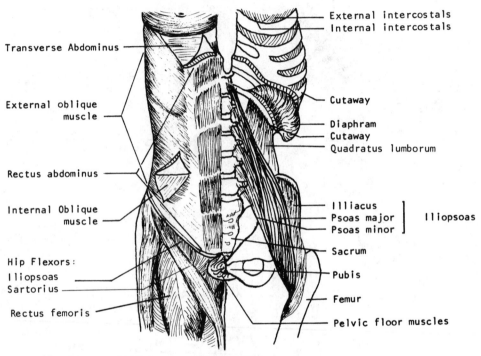

Transverse Abdominus

External oblique
muscle

Rectus abdominus

Internal Oblique
muscle

Hip Flexors:
Iliopsoas
Sartorius

Rectus femoris

External intercostals
Internal intercostals

Cutaway

Diaphram
Cutaway
Quadratus lumborum

Illiacus
Psoas major   Iliopsoas
Psoas minor

Sacrum

Pubis

Femur

Pelvic floor muscles

FIGURE 3.8(c)

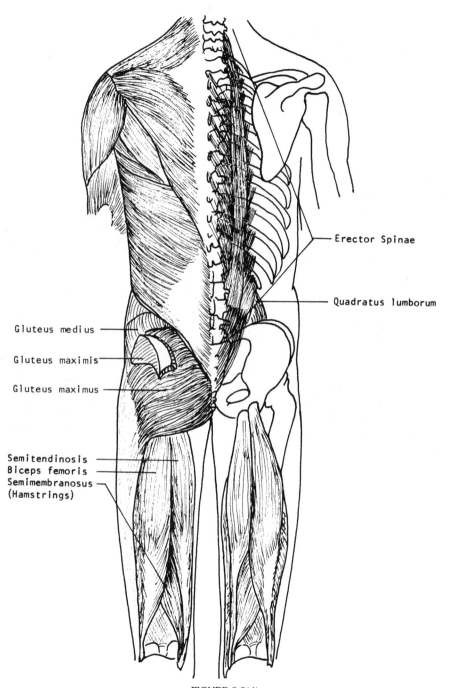

Erector Spinae

Quadratus lumborum

Gluteus medius

Gluteus maximis

Gluteus maximus

Semitendinosis
Biceps femoris
Semimembranosus
(Hamstrings)

FIGURE 3.8(d)

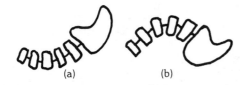

FIGURE 3.9

hind your head, and for a few minutes pretend you are at a disco. Rock and roll your pelvis gently, breathing with the movements. *Exhale* as your pelvis rotates backward flattening your back to the floor. *Inhale* as your pelvis tips forward, gently arching your lumbar spine (Figure 3.9A–B).

Your rock-and-roll movements are called tipping the pelvis forward, or toward the front of your body; tucking the pelvis backward, toward the back of your body. Now you are ready to move on to a relaxing and energizing exercise.

In the supine position, lying on your back, begin lifting and lowering your extended arms with your breath. As you inhale, your arms are lifting above you and then back behind you, parallel to, or touching, the floor. As you lift your extended arms, your rib cage expands and your lower back is in a relaxed secondary curve. Never force that curve! Your pelvis is relaxed in the tipped position. You are expanding for the breath like the opening of a bellows or an accordian. (See Figure 3.10A–C.) As you exhale, bring your

arms back beside you again. As they return to starting position your ribs relax. Your lower back presses to the floor and your pelvis is tucked. Buttocks, legs, and abdomen are all contracting and working to flatten your lumbar curve to the floor. (See Figure 3.11A.) This presses the air out of you just like a bellows. This is one cycle.

Points of Focus:

1. Do several cycles. Focus on your arms, spine, and breath moving freely and rhythmically together. Experience the *body* drawing the breath in and pressing the breath out. *Your body is breathing you.*

2. Keep your arms extended and moving together. In starting position, your palms are turned down. The arms rotate, palms turning toward each other, as you bring them above your head. Thumbs point toward the floor as your arms go back behind you.

3. Let your head relax and move freely with your arms and spine.

4. Keep knees in alignment with your hip joints and toes pointing straight ahead.

5. Press down evenly on the soles of your feet as you exhale. See how that helps you tuck your pelvis.

6. To tip, *relax* buttocks. To tuck, *contract* buttocks.

FIGURE 3.10

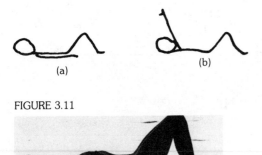

FIGURE 3.11

(a)

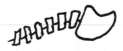

(b)

CAUTION: Guard against overarching your lumbar spine. Swaybacks need this tip. Look at the drawings in Figure 3.11B. Then inhale and bring your arms back behind you. Keep them there as you exhale and tuck your pelvis. Press your sacrum firmly to the floor, like a postage stamp to an envelope. Breathe smoothly and evenly as you hold the tuck. See how much curve you can take out of your lumbar spine. Now bring your arms down as you exhale. Relax. Your spine will feel long and alive, as though you'd been in traction.

Practice the Tip and Tuck, concentrating on the congruent movements of every part of your body, and you will understand a very powerful principle! You also have a foolproof way to energize and relax at the same time.

Table Tip and Tuck. Assume Table Pose, illustrated in Figure 3.12. Place your hands directly under your shoulder joints, your knees under your hip joints, thighs and shins forming a right angle. Your feet are in alignment with your knees. Toes point straight back, and soles of feet face upward. Your spine has the same curves as it did when you were lying on your back (supine). Even though you are turned over now, apply what you've learned in the supine position to this position. That's extrapolation!

Now gently tip and tuck your pelvis in Table Pose. Do several cycles. Keep your hips over your knees. Don't allow them to move back and forth. Just exhale and rotate your

FIGURE 3.12

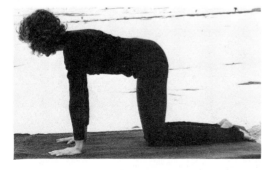

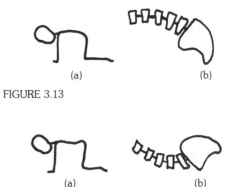

(a)   (b)

FIGURE 3.13

(a)   (b)

FIGURE 3-14

pelvis backward for the Tuck (Figure 3.13A—B). Inhale, rotating it forward for the Tip (Figure 3.14A—B).

If you have tight hamstrings, you may not be able to rotate your pelvis very much. If you have a swayback condition, you may rotate your pelvis too far forward. You have to be very aware of not overdoing it.

Then rest in Cat Stretch, by pushing your hips back to your heels and resting your extended arms on the floor in front of you. (See Figure 3.46.) If your knees can't take this position, place a rolled towel at the back of your knees to reduce the angle of flexion.

Cat-Cow Pose. When you are ready for the next step, assume Table Pose again. You will be doing the same thing you did in Table Pose, but this time your spine will flex and extend as you tip and tuck.

For Cat Pose, tuck your pelvis, drop your head, and round your back like an angry cat. Your hips (pelvis) are tucking and your spine is bending (flexing). This movement presses the air out of you, just like a bellows (Figure 3.15).

For Cow Pose, tip your pelvis, lift your head, and gently arch your upper back. The thoracic spine arches slightly as you draw your sternum forward (Figure 3.16). Do not overarch in the lumbar spine.

Move and breathe in a harmonious and relaxing rhythm. Do several cycles. Then

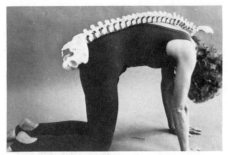

FIGURE 3.15

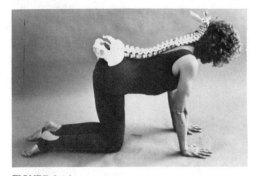

FIGURE 3.16

push your hips back again into Cat Stretch and relax. Process this very important pose. Cat-Cow is dynamite! Enjoy it. It relaxes and energizes.

CAUTION: Swaybacks, don't overarch your lumbar spine. Balance your pelvis. Draw your sternum forward so that your thoracic spine helps to draw your lumbar into extension. This is a *Two-Way Stretch*. Exercise restraint! *Find the balance between going too far and not far enough.*

Now you will use the Tip and Tuck principle in bending, lifting, and reaching. This is the Fulcrum-Lever Concept, which is based on the principle of a joint acting as a fulcrum. The surrounding bone or bones are the levers. Consider the pelvis and spine as a unit— the lever. The hip joints are the fulcrum. The pelvis and spine (lever) move on the hip joints (fulcrum). *Your spine will retain its stable S-curve as it follows the direction of the pelvis.* See Figure 3.17A–D.

Notice what happens as you use Tip and Tuck in the Fulcrum-Lever system to bend, lift, and reach.

Bending. Bending over can be misleading. It creates an image of the spine bending over. Think instead of the bend or flexion occurring at the fulcrum of the hip joints. The Fulcrum-Lever system makes it possible for your spine to retain its normal curves whenever possible and minimize overrounding of the back.

There are two basic ways of forward bending: Straight-Leg Forward Bend and Bent-Leg Forward Bend.

In order to do Straight-Leg Forward Bends and keep your legs straight, you have to be in excellent shape and be able to do Cosmic Sandwich very efficiently. You will see this 90° Forward Bend used often in Undercover Exercise. Most of the time, the arms are supported by a ledge of some kind, or one leg is forward in Split-Leg Forward Bend. (See Figure 3.18A—B.) This keeps some of the pressure off the lumbar spine and the lumbosacral joint, the joint where the last lumbar vertebra meets the sacrum.

If the arms do not help support the weight of the body, then you *must* undergird

FIGURE 3.18

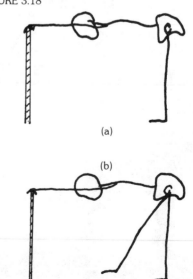

(a)

(b)

FIGURE 3.17

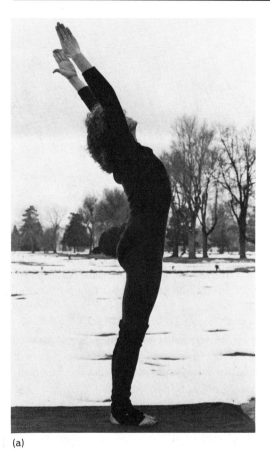

(a)

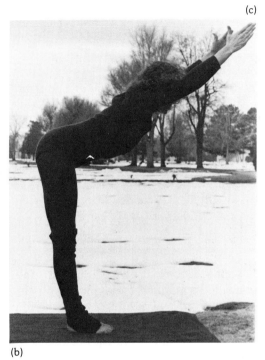

(c)

(b)

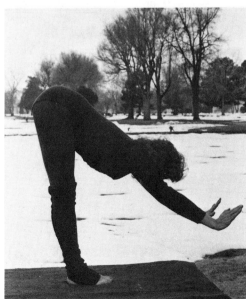

(c)

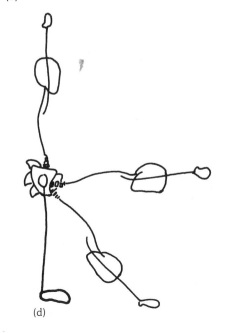

(d)

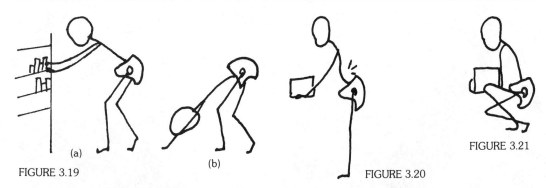

(a)

FIGURE 3.19

(b)

FIGURE 3.20

FIGURE 3.21

the spine with very strong abdominal muscles. *Never lift anything in this position!* Your abdominal and back muscles have all they can do to maintain and/or lift the body in this position.

CAUTION: If you do the Straight-Leg Forward Bends, you should have:

1. Hamstrings long enough to permit the pelvis to rotate to a balanced position.

2. Strong abdominal and pelvic-floor muscles to support the spine and keep pressure off the lumbosacral joint.

3. Place one leg forward to help support the weight of the torso (Split-Leg Forward Bend).

If you have any back problems or are not in top physical condition, use the Bent Leg Forward Bend (Figure 3.19A–B). Your flexed-knee position will help your abdominals support the spine.

KEY IDEA: For all forward bending, rotate your pelvis in a tipped or balanced position to keep your lower S-curve stable.

Lifting. For lifting, rotate your pelvis in the Tuck position while flexing your knees until you feel your lumbar curve flatten or straighten. This will protect the lower back from strain. If you are swaybacked and/or have back problems, the lumbar spine should be kept as flat and elongated as possible. That may mean that you have to tuck your pelvis and slightly round the lumbar in order to minimize your swayback.

If you use the Tip position while lifting, you will compress the lumbar discs and vertebrae (Figure 3.20). The Tuck position and Squat Pose enable you to lift, carry, and work with the spine in a more vertical position without strain to your lumbar region. You can use the Kneeling Squat, Half Squat, or Full Squat (Figure 3.21).

During your work or play, you may need to bend over (forward bend) from a squat or kneeling position. Use the Fulcrum-Lever Concept. (See Figure 3.22.) *Do not twist your back out of alignment while lifting or carrying.*

CAUTION: If you have stiff knees and/or hip joints, drop your tucked pelvis as much as your knees and hips will allow and use supports and aids whenever you can. Hold onto ledges, chairs, or walls (Figure 3.23). Your body has to compensate for any stiff joints that do not move easily.

Reaching Upward. For reaching, use the Tuck position of your pelvis and extend your

FIGURE 3.23

FIGURE 3.22

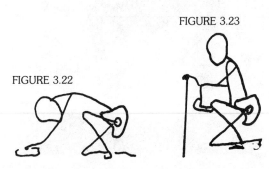

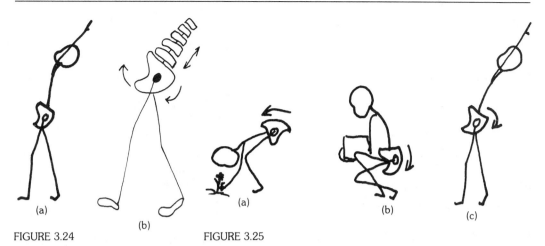

FIGURE 3.24   FIGURE 3.25

back as in Cow Pose. If you have to lean back a bit, the arching should come in the *thoracic,* not the lumbar, spine. Use your sternum to draw the spine up into extension so that there is no compression in the lower back. Dynamic Duo will help you learn to do this (Figure 3.24). One-Step Backbend in Configuration 7 teaches you to tuck your pelvis for reaching upward.

KEY IDEA: For the bending, lifting, and reaching you do every day, move the spine with the pelvis. The Tip and Tuck principle enables you to move your pelvis in a greater range of motion. The Fulcrum-Lever Concept enables you to move your spine in a safe and stable position.

In forward bending, rotate the pelvis forward in Tip position. In lifting or back-bending, rotate the pelvis backward in Tuck position. See Figure 3.25A—C.

Cosmic Sandwich You are now ready for the principle of Cosmic Sandwich, which trains you to keep the torso strong and evenly balanced supporting the primary and secondary curves of your spine.

Cosmic Sandwich got its name from a student who is a 74-year-old superman. He came up with the name in class one night while I was describing this principle as a peanut butter and jelly sandwich—the two slices of bread the frontal and back muscles, the filling your spine.

You have learned to support the spine in lifting, bending, and reaching. Cosmic Sandwich will teach you how to support your spine while sitting and standing. The asanas, or poses, to practice are Staff Pose, Back Press, and Mountain Pose.

SITTING CHECK-UP: Sit with your hips, back, and head against a wall. Extend your legs out in front of you. Can you get your hips to the wall? Can you get your hips to the wall but not your lower back? Can you touch your head to the wall?

If you can't get your hips to the wall, you have tight hamstring muscles. Tight hamstrings act as a vise on your pelvis, keeping it from rotating freely. A firm cushion or folded blanket under your hips will help you rotate your pelvis and safely lengthen your hamstrings. Scoot your hips all the way to the wall

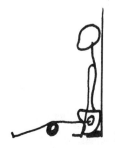

FIGURE 3.26

and then feel as if your hips are rolling forward off the support (Figure 3.26). This will rotate your pelvis from a tucked position to a more balanced position.

If you can't get your lower back to the wall, you have a swayback. To help correct this, flex your knees and bring them toward your chest, soles of feet resting on the floor. Notice how easily your back presses against the wall. Your pelvis is rotated backward and your back muscles are relaxed. Now slide your feet away from your hips until your lower back begins to arch away from the wall. If your legs do not completely straighten, place a rolled towel under your knees.

If you can't get your head to the wall, you have a rounded middle or upper back and probably a turkey neck. Place a tightly rolled face towel between your shoulder blades to lift the thoracic spine and open your chest. Now you're ready for Staff Pose.

Staff Pose (Dandasana). Think of yourself as a right angle. (See Figure 3.27.) Press your back against a wall or sit away from the wall with your legs extended along the floor. Place your arms at your sides, palms down beside your hips. Make your spine tall and your legs long. In the beginning you may need to use your aids to assume the right-angle position. (Look again at Figure 3.26.)

FIGURE 3.27

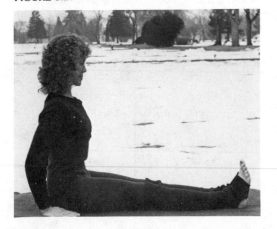

Points of Focus:
1. Legs hip-width apart.
2. Flex feet, drawing your toes upward.
3. Contract your thigh muscles (quadriceps).
4. Balance your pelvis.
5. Be a Cosmic Sandwich.
6. Relax shoulders and arms, palms down on the floor.
7. Chin parallel to the floor.
8. Eyes straight ahead, soft and clear.
9. Breathe evenly and rhythmically (Rhythmical Complete Breathing, Chapter 2).
10. Practice a Two-Way Stretch—as gravity pulls you downward, use it as an anchor to extend upward.

CAUTIONS:

1. If your knees hyperextend (knee joints lock backward), place a rolled towel under your knees.
2. If your hamstrings or sciatic nerves send you pain signals, *stop.* Keep your knees flexed. Gradually you'll be able to extend your legs with practice.
3. If you have a rounded thoracic curve, draw your shoulder blades together.
4. If you have a swayback condition, *do not* draw your shoulder blades together. You'll end up with "chicken ribs." Instead, contract your abdominal muscles. Imagine that your abdominals can draw your pubic bone and lower ribs together. This will help balance your pelvis.

Now turn Staff Pose upside down (Figure 3.28). Lie on your side in a fetal position and scoot your hips to the wall. Turn over on your back, bend your knees, and place your feet on the wall. This is a much more relaxing way to practice Staff Pose. Great for the 4:00 P.M. blahs! Very relaxing and comforting for your tired legs and feet after a long, long day.

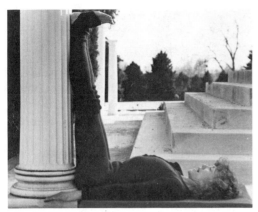

FIGURE 3.28

Do a few Tip and Tucks with smooth and even breathing. Then gradually extend your legs, resting them on the wall. If your lower back arches or you have sciatic problems, keep your knees bent. (See Figure 3.29.)

STANDING CHECK-UP: Standing isn't easy because our feet are a very narrow base. Even the broadest bodies still have the same narrow base. We are like a pop bottle turned upside down. Mountain Pose teaches us to capitalize on the base we've got . . . no matter how small.

Remember how you checked your primary and secondary curves while lying on the floor and sitting against the wall? Run the same check standing with your back against a wall.

Stand with your feet a few inches from the wall. Your ankles should be aligned directly under your hip joints. First check the curves of your spine in standing position. *Start from the ground up.* Feel the curve of your

FIGURE 3.29

sacrum against the wall. Now place your hand between the wall and your lumbar curve. How much space do you have there? Do you have more or less space now than when you were lying down? Follow your spine upward into your thoracic curve. Is it a rounded, a flattened, or a normal curve? Now check your cervical curve. How far from the wall is it? Does your head touch the wall or is it difficult to get the back of your head against the wall?

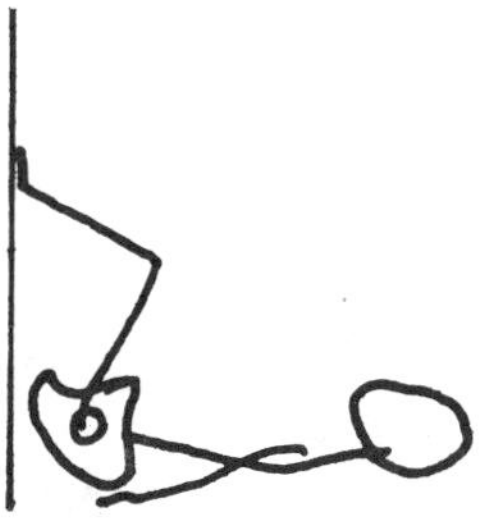

Now practice the Tip and Tuck of your pelvis against the wall, just as you did on the floor. These rocks and rolls show you again what happens to your pelvis and lower back when you tip and tuck. If you stand or walk with your pelvis in Tip position, you create a swayback. A Tuck position flattens your lower back and usually creates a tight butt and flexed knees. *For an elegant stance and an attractive walk, you need a balanced pelvis.*

Back Press. Here's an excellent exercise to give you that! You'll use it over and over again to rest your tired back. Swaybacks, this is your gold mine!

Stand against the wall with your feet 12 inches away from the wall. Bend your knees and slide your hips downward until you can firmly press your lower back against the wall. Hold that position. Feel your lower back lengthen, your abdominal and thigh muscles contract. Keep your hips above the level of your knees. See Figure 3.30.

This is just like the Staff Pose at the wall. Increase the difficulty of flattening your lower back to the wall by lifting your arms above your head. Hold the position, working your abdominals to lengthen your back. Now slide your hips upward and relax, supported by the wall. Step away from the wall and see how much easier it is to stand with your *pelvis balanced* as in Cosmic Sandwich.

You used abdominal muscles to get the Tuck position in the Back Press. This gives you a balanced pelvis without the tight butt. It's also a great exercise to train your body for walking, standing, or moving gracefully.

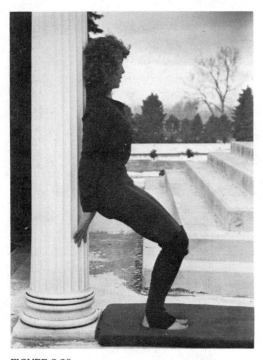

FIGURE 3.30

A balanced pelvis is essential to beautiful posture. You've seen the effects of an out-of-balance pelvis: the backside waving like a flag in swayback or dropped like an elephant's behind in the slump! It takes tremendous physical and emotional work to give up postures that reflect old habits. Mountain Pose helps us deal with our posture as a picture of how we think and feel about ourselves.

Mountain Pose (Tadasana). Apply everything you've learned in Cosmic Sandwich to this elegant and rewarding pose, shown in Figure 3.31A–B. It will form the foundation of your walking posture. Don't be surprised if Mountain Pose feels unnatural at first. Old habits get to feeling very natural, and change may feel very unnatural! We make changes only when we're ready! I remember one student, a lawyer, who absolutely hated practicing the Mountain Pose until she discovered that it was changing her image in the courtroom.

Here's the way to assume Mountain Pose:

1. *Plant your feet.* Create a broad and firm base, like a mountain. Let your body ascend upward out of its base, a mountain peak rising into the clouds. Point your toes straight ahead. Make sure that the insides of your feet are parallel to each other or feet together. Make your base very, very firm, distributing the weight evenly over the soles of your feet. Lift up through your arches. Relax the tension at the back of your knees. Extend the knee joint by grounding (planting) your heels in a downward direction and lifting your thighs in an upward direction. Your kneecaps will lift as you firm your thighs. If you tend to hyperextend your knees, flex the knees slightly.

2. *Balance your pelvis.* Think of your pelvic girdle as a bowl full of cherries. Don't tilt it forward or back. Balance it!

3. *Lift your sternum.* Create space between the shoulder blades by expanding your rib cage to the front, back, and sides. Your rib cage will feel like a beehive.

4. *Relax your shoulders.* Let your arms hang loosely from your shoulder joints.

5. *Center your head.* Lift upward from the base of your skull. The chin is at right angles to the throat and the gaze is straight ahead. Picture yourself hanging by the top of your head from an imaginary skyhook.

6. *Keep growing upward.* Stand erect and tall as a mountain.

Dynamic Duo The third of the Big Three Principles builds on the first two. Dynamic Duo uses Cosmic Sandwich muscle balancing and teaches you how to do a backbend without overarching the lower back. Why would you want to do a backbend? So that you can reach up or backward without damaging your spine. Your spine was meant to bend forward,

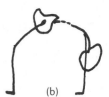

FIGURE 3.32

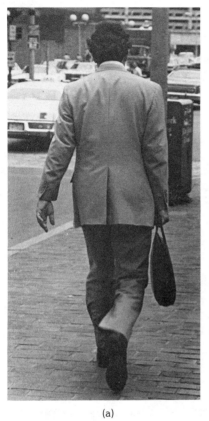

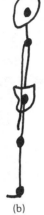

(a)   (b)

FIGURE 3.31

your back even while backbending (Figure 3.32A–B). You'll practice Coffee Break Stretch, Cobra, and Desk Pose to learn this principle.

KEY IDEA: The difference between Cosmic Sandwich and Dynamic Duo is that in Cosmic Sandwich, *you are keeping your pelvis balanced.* In Dynamic Duo, *you have to tuck your pelvis or the lever will bend too much in the lower back.*

Coffee Break Stretch. Look at Figure 3.33, and then let's find out what happens when

FIGURE 3.33

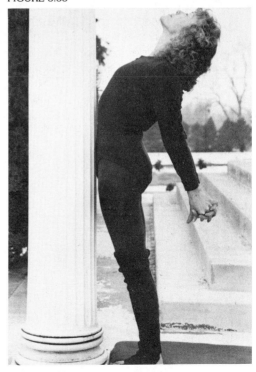

backward, and side to side. Full range of movement gives you many, many more options for positioning and maneuvering your body in a safe and powerful way.

You've just learned how to support your spine in the everyday positions of bending, lifting, reaching, sitting, and standing. But backbending is a challenge. It is a movement that is so poorly understood and painful for most people that very early in life we learn to avoid it. Professional dancers and gymnasts are among the few who are trained to do backbends. Now you can have the same training.

When you think of a backbend, you probably get a picture of acrobats making their backs into deep V curves. Dynamic Duo enables you to lengthen the lumbar curve of you try to do a simple backbend. Imagine that you've been working at your desk for several hours and you need to stretch. Stand up in Mountain Pose. Get yourself aligned and centered as you did in Cosmic Sandwich. Now stretch your arms back behind you, clasp your hands, and stretch. If you have difficulty clasping hands because of tight shoulders, grasp a tie or belt between your hands.

What's good about this stretch? Possibly nothing at the moment. Just trying to get your arms behind your back may be difficult for you right now! You may find your ribs protruding (chicken ribs), lumbar curve exaggerated, and pelvis out of alignment. On the other hand, your chest may have collapsed, shoulders rounded, cervical curve exaggerated (turkey neck), and you are leaning forward with a rounded lower back. How can you create Cosmic Sandwich with your arms behind your back?

Find an empty wall space and stand facing the wall, toes pointing straight ahead. If you keep your pelvis balanced or tipped and try to reach backward, the lever (pelvis-spine) will bend. And where does it bend? Right in the lower back, causing compression to discs and nerves. Instead, tuck your pelvis to lengthen your lower back (Figure 3.34A–B).

Now, the problem is that there's a natural limit to how far the pelvis can rotate in

Tuck position. You are limited by the structure of the joints and the condition of your muscles, tendons, and ligaments. The muscles in the groin that flex or bend the hips are called *hip flexors*. Because your pelvis is flexed more often than extended, these muscles are usually short. Shortened hip flexors keep the pelvis in a tipped position, causing a swayback. That's why Dynamic Duo is so important. (Look again at Figure 3.8, parts A and C.)

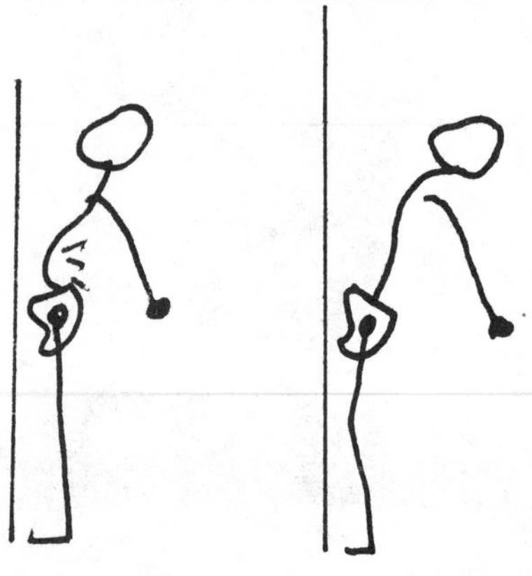

When you practice tucking your pelvis to its extreme Tuck position, you are lengthening the hip flexors; doing that permits your lumbar spine to elongate as much as possible. Now with that understanding, let's see what you can do to make the Coffee Break Stretch invigorating *and* safe for your back.

As you stretch your arms behind you, tuck your pelvis. Press your pubic bone toward the wall. The hip flexors have to stretch to permit this backward rotation of the pelvis and extension of the hips. Your abdominals contract to pull your pubic bone forward, and your lower back elongates.

Clasping your hands, lift your extended arms straight back and upward. Expand your chest, arching your thoracic spine upward. Feel as if your sternum is being drawn upward by that imaginary skyhook. Keep your head balanced and don't allow it to drop backward.

There you are. A Coffee Break Stretch every bit as invigorating as a cup of coffee, but no coffee nerves! Step away from the wall and do the stretch without the wall to help you. Now practice the same principle lying face downward on the floor.

Cobra Pose (Bhujangasana). Lie down on the floor in prone position (on your abdomen) with a mat or carpet under you. Place your hands, palms down, over your buttocks. Do a few pelvic rocks and rolls. Notice how tipping your pelvis forward increases your lumbar curve and compresses your spine. Now tuck your pelvis backward, pressing your pubic bone to the floor. See how much you can extend or elongate your lumbar spine.

FIGURE 3.34

(a)   (b)

KEY IDEA: Knowing how much you need to tuck your pelvis to elongate your lumbar curve is crucial to any backbending movement.

Now place a folded pad or firm pillow, two to three inches thick, under your abdomen. Make it only as wide as the space between the lower ribs and the upper rim of the pelvis. You want to be able to press the pubic bone down to the floor without the pillow getting in the way.

Relax your arms next to your body. As you exhale, rotate your pelvis backward into a tucked position. Press the pubic bone down into the mat or carpet. Can you feel the lumbar spine elongating? Good! The pillow or pad under your abdomen lifts the lumbar spine a bit and keeps it from arching. This aid is a *must* for all swaybacks!

Now exhale and see how much you can straighten the lumbar curve using your gluteal muscles to tuck the pelvis. Exhale again, and this time relax your gluteal muscles and use your abdominal muscles to help tuck the pelvis. Keep your buttocks as relaxed as possible. You probably found it much easier to elongate the lumbar spine by using your gluteal muscles. Most people find it difficult to use their abdominal muscles in the prone position. And if they do use their abdominals, it's usually by pushing the abdomen out with exertion or effort. But there's a better way! You can get an elevator effect by using your deep abdominal muscles together with the powerful pelvic floor muscles to assist the gluteals. These are your *core muscles*. (Look again at Figure 3.8C.)

Learn to use the Pelvic Floor Pull-Ups by imagining that you have to go to the bathroom but can't find one. See section on Core Power: Pelvic Floor Pull-Ups (Chapter 3 Back Trainers). Hold on . . . with *core power!* This is a subtle but extremely powerful undergirding principle. Exhaling, pull those pelvic floor and abdominal muscles up and in. They are your undercover strength and vitality.

Now exhale, using this core power to lift

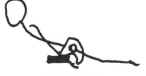

FIGURE 3.35

your shoulders, head, and chest off the floor like a cobra spreading his hood. Hold this position for a few cycles of breathing and notice what muscles you're using to lift your torso. Then exhaling, return to prone position and relax. See Figure 3.35.

Often, only buttock and back muscles are used when practicing back-strengthening exercises prescribed by doctors, physical therapists, and back-care classes. It's the common way of exercising. When you try to strengthen your back without incorporating Dynamic Duo, you can easily overarch and compress the lumbar spine. So how have you helped yourself?

The secret of support and lift is using the powerful balance of your abdominal and pelvic floor muscles in combination with your gluteal, leg, and back muscles. Practicing Dynamic Duo is the safest way to strengthen your back. Once you've learned it, you've got the polish and poise of a well-trained dancer or athlete.

Chest Expansion in Cobra. Now practice the same undercover lift in this variation of Cobra Pose, which is like Coffee Break Stretch lying face downward. See Figure 3.36. Clasp your hands behind your back, just as you did

FIGURE 3.36

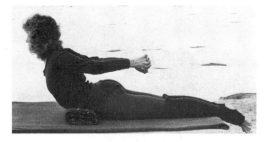

in the Coffee Break Stretch. Your hands are resting on your buttocks, thumbs downward. Use a tie if you can't clasp your hands. The backward stretch of your arms has expanded your ribs, and you may already feel your back muscles contracting with some compression in the small of your back. Exhale and tuck your pelvis. Use Core Power! Is your lumbar spine elongated?

Now inhale and get set—arms straight and hands clasped over buttocks, forehead down, pelvis tucked, and legs extended and firm. Exhale and use Dynamic Duo to lift your torso. Simultaneously draw your arms and hands back over your buttocks. Your breathing will quicken as you hold the pose. Concentrate on elongating the lumbar spine as you exhale. Hold the pose for several breaths, and then lower the body on an exhalation. Relax.

Desk Pose (Variation of Setu Bandha). Turn over on your back and align your body as you did for Supine Tip and Tuck. Desk Pose is like the Chest Expansion in Cobra, except that now the back of your body is the base instead of your front. (See Figure 3.37.) This practice of extrapolation helps you to sharpen your wits and adapt to change. Exhale and lift your hips just an inch off the floor (Figure 3.38). Notice the abdominals, buttocks, and thighs working together. This position is the "miracle worker" for lower back strain and pain. Breathe smoothly and hold the Tuck position as long as you can. Then slowly allow your buttocks to return to the floor. Relax.

FIGURE 3.37

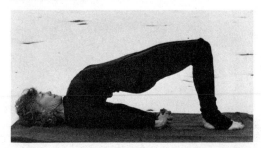

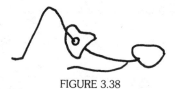

FIGURE 3.38

CAUTION: If you have back problems, don't lift your hips any higher than an inch off the floor. Keep your waistline on the floor. Hold the position tucking the pelvis giving your back a chance to stretch out. Create a feeling of traction in your lower back (Figure 3.38).

For more work in the pose, lift your tucked pelvis as if a crane above you were cradling your hips in a sling, lifting them up and up an inch at a time. Press down on your arms, hands, and inside edges of your feet. Keep your knees and feet in alignment with the hip joints. With every exhalation, visualize the crane lifting your pelvis off the floor another inch. Lift until you feel your lumbar spine beginning to arch. Stop there. Hold the pose, firmly tucking your pelvis to elongate your lumbar spine.

Use Dynamic Duo to tuck your tail and keep your spine long and strong. As you practice, your hip flexors will stretch and your core muscles will become more powerful. You will be able to lift higher and keep your lumbar spine elongated.

When you feel that you are balanced and strong in this part of the pose, you may go on. Clasp your hands together on the floor just as you did in the Coffee Break Stretch and Chest Expansion in Cobra. (See Figure 3.37.)

Points of Focus
1. Feel your shoulders roll back and downward, making cushions beneath you.
2. Your arms are extended and firm, fingers clasped.
3. Your chest expands and your shoulder blades move together. Draw your lower ribs inward. Use your abdominals.

4. Your breathing quickens as you work for balanced strength in the pose.

5. Keep the buttocks and legs firm. With every exhalation, lift the pelvis and elongate the entire spinal column.

KEY IDEA: Use Dynamic Duo and your core power to keep the front and back of your body muscularly balanced, to tuck your pelvis as far as possible, stretch your hip flexors, and keep the pelvis-spine lever elongated and strong.

Have you noticed that you have been doing the same work while standing in the Coffee Break Stretch, lying on your stomach in Cobra, and lying on your back in Desk Pose? Each time the principles are the same. The *pull of gravity on the body* is the only thing that changes. As your body position changes, different muscles have to work a little harder or a little less to acommodate the change. The Cobra Pose and Coffee Break Stretch are easier because gravity is helping you to tuck your pelvis. In Desk Pose, you are tucking your pelvis *and* lifting your body *against* the pull of gravity.

No matter what position you're in, whether you are right side up or upside down, the Big Three Principles are yours to apply. Your body is like a finely tuned instrument and you're learning how to play it, no matter what position you're in.

KEY IDEA: It takes consistent and persistent practice to train the front muscles of your body and the back muscles of your body to work together as a *Dynamic Duo*. It's division of labor. No one muscle group carries the load alone!

Now you are ready for the other Back Trainers. You can use the Big Three Principles—Tip and Tuck, Cosmic Sandwich, and Dynamic Duo—to give you the essentials—circulation, alignment, and extension. The rest of the Back Trainers will give you practice in applying your understanding of these principles. And what do *you* get out

of it? Those priceless commodities—good health, good looks, and good humor.

Listen to what your body tells you and practice the Back Trainers at the level you feel most comfortably challenged. There is always some discomfort in challenge. Decide just how much challenge you need. Make sure that you are not pushing yourself too hard, hurrying, or resisting growth. Move slowly, allowing time for your body to tell you about itself. You have a built-in biofeedback system. Pay attention to its signals. Even the simplest movements offer incredible challenges in awareness and understanding.

Undercover Exercise is not just something you do, but a process of understanding what you do.

Knee-to-Chest Series   This series gently lengthens back muscles and hamstrings, strengthens abdominal muscles, relaxes, and energizes. It is good for easing back discomfort and aiding digestion.

CAUTION: If you have back or sciatic nerve problems, do this series with both legs bent. As your condition improves, you can keep one leg extended in the exercises.

Knee-to-Chest Squeeze (Apanasana). See Figure 3.39A–B.

- Lie down in alignment on your back (supine position).

FIGURE 3.39

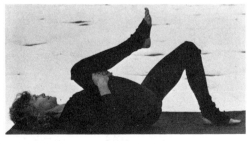

(a)

(b)

- Exhaling, bend one knee and draw it toward your chest. Keep the opposite leg straight or bent.
- Place your hands between the thigh and calf of your bent leg.
- On every exhalation, squeeze the bent knee to your chest.
- On every inhalation, relax. Keep the leg flexed as you squeeze and release.
- Continue this slow rhythmical breathing, squeezing and relaxing.
- Your back and one leg are your base. Keep your awareness on your base, as well as the moving leg.
- Change legs and repeat the exercise.
- Vary the exercise by holding the bent knee close to your chest as you breathe rhythmically.

Supine One-Legger (Variation of Supta Padangusthasana). See Figure 3.40.

- Lie on your back.
- Exhaling, draw one knee upward until your thigh bone is perpendicular to the floor, your shin and thigh bone form a 90° angle.
- Hold onto your leg at the back of your thigh, arms extended.
- Keep your lower back pressed firmly to the floor.
- Keep your foot flexed.
- Use a tie around the ball of your foot. Grasp the ends of the tie with both hands. Press your heel upward and gradually straighten your leg (Figure 3.41).
- Keep your upper arms close to your sides. Head and shoulders remain relaxed on the floor.
- Gently stretch your hamstrings and achilles tendon (back of heel).
- Release the tie and bend your knee, hugging the leg to your chest.
- Extend the leg on the floor and relax.

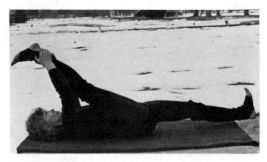

FIGURE 3.40

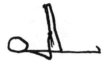

FIGURE 3.41

- Notice the length of the leg that you just stretched compared to the other leg. Doesn't it feel longer?
- Change legs and repeat.
- Then do the exercise grasping the back of the leg instead of the tie.
- Caution: For tight hamstrings or sciatic problems, keep your knee bent and just gently press the heel upward as you exhale.

Head to Knee. See Figure 3.42 A–B.

- Lie on your back.
- Exhaling, draw one knee to your chest.
- Inhale and then exhale drawing your head toward your knee.
- Keep your shoulders level and drawn away from your ears.
- Breathe quietly as you use your abdominal muscles to keep the torso flexed.
- Exhaling, lower your head and shoulders.
- Relax.
- Repeat with opposite leg bent.
- Continue until your abdominal muscles feel "warm."
- Keep your head to your knee by rolling the upper back off the floor. This will

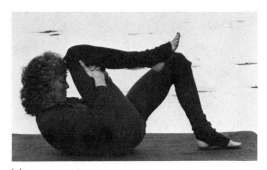

(a)

(b)

FIGURE 3.42

contract your abdominal muscles and make them work against the pull of gravity.

Huggy Pose. See Figure 3.43.

- Lying on your back, bring both knees to your chest.
- Grasp the backs of your thighs.
- Exhaling, draw your thighs as close to your chest as you can.
- Keep your head and shoulders relaxed on the floor.
- Inhale and relax the squeeze. Exhale and squeeze.

FIGURE 3.43

FIGURE 3.44

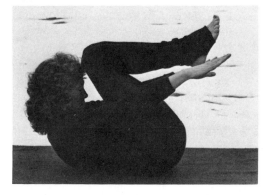

- Repeat the squeeze-relax movements in a smooth, rhythmical pattern.
- On the next exhalation, draw your head to your knees.
- To increase the difficulty, stretch your arms toward the wall in front of you. See Figure 3.44.
- Keep your shoulders level and drawn away from your ears.
- Breathe for several cycles while your abdominals vigorously work to hold that position.
- Exhaling, relax on the floor with your knees close to your chest.
- Slide your legs out and relax.
- Repeat until your abdominals feel warm.

Turkey Pose. See Figure 3.45.

- This is a take-off on Huggy Pose. Begin in the same position.
- Instead of keeping your knees together, separate them, drawing the legs and feet as far apart as possible. Now you know how this pose got its name—you'll look like a Thanksgiving turkey rather than a live one.
- Exhaling, draw your knees toward your shoulder joints.
- Inhaling, release the squeeze moving your legs away from your chest until your arms straighten.

FIGURE 3.45

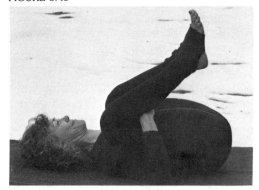

- Continue these gentle squeeze-relax movements with your breathing for 5 to 20 cycles.
- On your next exhalation, hold the squeeze.
- Slowly let your legs slide out and relax. This is the best exercise in the world for a sore and/or tired back! Use it.

Cat Stretch. See Figure 3.46.

- Sit on your heels.
- Rest your torso on your thighs, arms extending out in front of you on the floor. Your head rests on the floor or a cushion.
- Point your feet straight back behind you. If your feet hurt in this position, place some padding under your ankles to ease the stretch; your feet will gradually accommodate the stretch.
- Stretch your fingers and arms like a cat sharpening its claws.
- Stretch from toes to fingers.
- Relax your shoulders, drawing them away from your ears.

Child's Pose (Darnikasana). See Figure 3.47.

- From Cat Stretch bring your arms beside your thighs, turning palms up. This is the same position as Huggy Pose, except that now your body weight is on your legs and feet. You can place a pillow or rolled towel between your thighs and calves if your legs are very uncomfortable.
- Relax your head, shoulders, and arms.
- Breathe quietly for a few cycles as you rest in this peaceful pose.

Core Power This series develops abdominal and pelvic-floor muscles. These are the core muscles that enable you to do Cosmic Sandwich and Dynamic Duo. The Trainers begin gently and increase in difficulty. Even the first two are easy but powerful exercises. Practice them until you can proceed with the

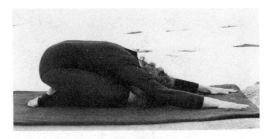

FIGURE 3.46

     FIGURE 3.47

others. Your secret code to back strength is *core power!*

CAUTION: Remember to flatten your abdominals as you exhale. Instead of "pooching" them out like a dome, draw them gently in toward your spine. There is a feeling of strength and support in the abdominals rather than one of tension and hardness.

Neck Press. See Figure 3.48.

- Lie down on your back *in alignment.*
- Bend both knees, and place the soles of your feet on the floor. Your knees and feet are in line with your hip joints.
- Remember how you tipped and tucked your pelvis in Tip and Tuck? Do the same with your head.
- Inhaling, tip your chin upward. This increases the cervical curve.
- Exhaling, tuck your chin down and inward, pressing down on the back of your neck. This extends and elongates the cervical curve.
- If you have a "turkey neck," your chin will already be tipped upward. Concentrate on tucking, rather than tipping, your chin. Remember to use a small pillow or pad under your head.
- Repeat the pressing and releasing of

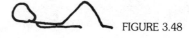   FIGURE 3.48

FIGURE 3.49

your neck, holding each press for several breaths. This is great to relieve tension headaches.

Head Roll-Up. See Figure 3.49.

- Assume the Neck Press position.
- Exhaling, roll your head and shoulders off the floor.
- Keep your shoulders and arms drawn toward your hips. Don't hunch your shoulders.
- Feel your abdominal muscles contracting maximally. Breathe quietly, and hold this position until your body says enough.
- Exhale, returning your shoulders and head to the floor. Relax.
- Start with one Head Roll-Up and then gradually increase in number and/or time duration for each one.

Torso Curls. See Figure 3.50.

- Assume the Neck Press position with your lower legs on a chair seat or your feet pressed against a wall, legs bent at 90° angle.
- Fold your arms over your chest.
- Exhaling, curl your head and torso off the floor. Keep your shoulders and elbows reaching toward your hips.
- Breathe quietly, feeling your abdominals working, getting warmer and warmer and warmer!
- Exhaling, uncurl and return to the floor. Relax.
- Repeat several times.
- Vary the abdominal work by reaching diagonally across your torso (Figure 3.51).

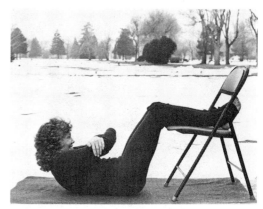

FIGURE 3.50

FIGURE 3.51

FIGURE 3.52

Sit-Back. See Figure 3.52.

- Sit in Staff Pose.
- Bend your knees and rest the soles of your feet on the floor.
- Grasp the back of your thighs.
- Exhale, and lift your feet a few inches off the floor. Hold and breathe in Cosmic Sandwich.
- Let go of your thighs and extend your arms like oars beside your knees, palms toward knees and thumbs up.
- Hold here, breathing quietly. Work your abdominal and back muscles equally in Cosmic Sandwich.
- Exhale, and return to starting position.

Boat Pose (Paripurna Navasana). See Figure 3.53.

- Sit with your knees bent, the soles of your feet on the floor. Knees are in line with hip joints.
- Place your hands, palms down, beside or slightly in front of your hips.

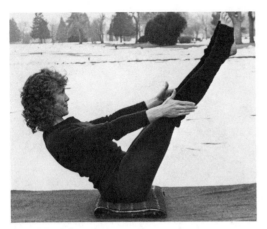

FIGURE 3.53

- Then lean back and balance on your sit bones, as in Sit Back.
- Exhale, and lift one leg higher than the level of your head. Keep the leg extended (Figure 3.54).

    FIGURE 3.54

- Balance your pelvis. Become a Cosmic Sandwich.
- Exhale, and return your foot to the floor.
- Repeat, extending the opposite leg.
- Now lift both legs simultaneously.
- Keeping your Cosmic Sandwich, exhale and lift your hands and arms to the oar position.
- Hold this position as you breathe rhythmically.
- Exhale and return feet to floor. Phhh!
- Relax.

Pelvic Floor Pull-Ups.

- Lie on the floor in supine position.
- Exhale and tuck your pelvis in Tuck position. Breathe rhythmically as you press your pelvis down to the floor.

Imagine the pull of gravity drawing your rectum and/or vagina toward your lower back.

- Squeeze firmly on those inner canals of your body. The muscles in that area are unfamiliar to most people.
- Use your powers of extrapolation here. Imagine that you are holding a gauge that measures the strength of your grip. As your hand closes around the gauge, it measures your grip strength.
- Think of this same gauge testing the grip strength of your rectum and/or vagina. As your squeeze or pull in your pelvic-floor muscles, the gauge measures your grip strength.
- Now that you have the idea, squeeze and release, squeeze and release. This is a vital part of your Core Power!
- Do Pelvic Floor Pull-Ups in Staff Pose against the wall or in a Squat position (Figure 3.55A—B).

     FIGURE 3.55

(a)   (b)

Squats These techniques bring a rich blood supply to the pelvic area and improve sluggish bowels, helping with waste elimination. They increase flexibility in hips, knees, and ankles, as well as strengthen legs and ease back tension.

CAUTION: If you have knee or ankle problems, go down into a squat only as far as you comfortably can. Hold onto a support at all times to minimize the weight on knees and ankles and to help balance yourself. If you can't go down into a squat right now, practice the Turkey Pose until your knees and/or ankles can accommodate the squat.

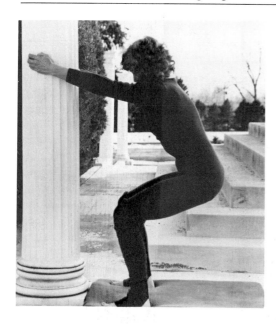

FIGURE 3.56

Doorknob Squat. See Figure 3.56.

- Stand in Mountain Pose.
- Straddle the open edge of a door. Grasp both doorknobs with your hands. You can use a pole or column, as shown in Figure 3.56.
- Position your feet so that they are wider than hip-width apart. Toes are pointing straight ahead, if possible.
- Lean outward from the door, extending your arms.
- Exhaling, slowly lower your hips to just above your knees.
- Hang out there, breathing rhythmically.
- Balance your pelvis. Some of you will have to tuck, others tip to do this.
- Lower your hips as far as you comfortably can (Figure 3.57).

FIGURE 3.57

- Hang in traction as gravity pulls your pelvis downward.
- Press your feet firmly to the floor and return to standing position.
- Repeat rhythmically according to your ability. It's fun.

Bellows Squat. See Figure 3.58.

CAUTION: Practice this squat only if you can comfortably go all the way down in Doorknob Squat.

- Stand in Mountain Pose.
- Exhaling, lower your hips toward the floor. Tuck your pelvis as you go down.
- If you need to, hold onto a ledge or door for balance.
- Place your elbows and upper arms to the inside of your knees. Bring your hands together in prayer position.
- Inhaling, push your knees apart with your elbows, opening like a bellows.
- Exhaling, bring your knees together, pressing your arms between your legs, closing like a bellows.
- Do as many cycles as you feel comfortable doing.

FIGURE 3.58

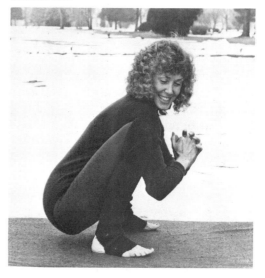

- Exhaling, tuck your pelvis and stand erect.

Easy Back Twist This technique releases tension in the back and shoulders, and increases shoulder and neck mobility. It actually massages the abdominal organs and lymph glands. See Figure 3.59.

- Lie on your back in alignment.
- Stretch your arms in *T* position on the floor.
- Bend your left knee and place your left foot on top of your right knee.
- Grasp your left knee with your right hand.
- Exhaling, draw your left knee toward the floor, rolling onto your right hip. Keep your right leg firmly extended.
- Roll your head to the left and look over your left shoulder. Stretch your left arm along the floor to a two o'clock position. If your arm does not rest on the floor, place a cushion under it. Breathe and stretch.
- Change legs, and twist to the opposite side.
- Roll back to center, align your body, and relax.

You have just finished the Back Trainers. You have had the opportunity to practice and apply the Big Three Principles, an undercover revolution. They represent a turning point. Through them, you are breaking away from past uptightness in body and mind to a new sense of poise and energy in your work and play. Relish the new length and catlike suppleness of your body.

FIGURE 3.59

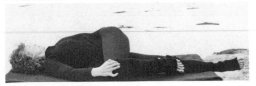

BODY TRAINERS

The Back Trainers have given you a solid foundation. Body Trainers are designed to build a great house on that foundation. Everyday life will offer you endless opportunities to apply what you've learned and to strengthen and extend yourself.

Body Trainers are organized into easy-to-remember configurations. Each configuration is a group of poses, or body positions, similar in shape. Program the shapes in your body-mind computer as you practice them daily. Then, in life situations you can call up an appropriate Undercover Exercise.

Shapes within the configurations are like pieces of a jigsaw puzzle. You can turn them upside down and switch them all around to see where they fit into your life. Dog Stretch is upside down Boat Pose. The 90° Forward Bend is Staff Pose turned on end (Figure 3.60). You can lean on the counter and do a 90° Forward Bend at the supermarket. At home you can turn it around and do the Dog Stretch while looking for that lost shoe in the closet. If you're restricted from poses that place your head lower than your heart, Intense Forward Bend is out for you. Well, just turn it around and do Supine Jack Knife or Seated Forward Bend.

There are no excuses in Undercover Exercise. Ask your doctor, physical therapist, or trainer to give you tips that will adapt your workout to your own personal specifications. Go shopping among these configurations, looking through the figures in each configuration to pick the ones that you can *safely* practice.

How to Practice

Directions For simplicity, the directions are given for one side only. Be sure to practice the other side as well. If you find yourself spending more time on the right side than the left, start with the left side next time. Most people

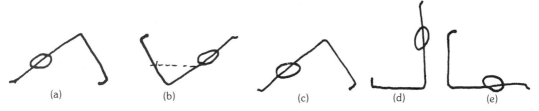

FIGURE 3.60

spend more time practicing the first side longer than the second. Once you know which side is dominant, practice the *less* dominant side first.

Breath   Allow your breathing to adapt rhythmically to the demands of the exercise. Forward bends are quieting, and your breath will become long and rhythmical. Backbends and twists are envigorating and demand more oxygen. Your breath will quicken. Listen to your body. Your breathing will naturally adapt to the needs of your body, if you allow it to. "Breathe quietly" means letting your breath be natural and spontaneous.

Your inhalations are "enablers." Use them to get set. Your exhalations are your "movers." Use them to extend, elongate, and work. As a general practice, make your exhalations longer than your inhalations. This will help stabilize the acid-base balance in your body while you work. No Puff . . . puff . . . puffing. Choo choo train breath is for trains.

You will often find breathing directions for exhaling and not inhaling. Please inhale after each exhalation. It'll help you stay alive!

Base   Every pose has a base. The parts of your body that come in contact with the floor form this base.

Adjustments   Fix it from the ground up. Adjustments need to begin at the base, or your foundation. If the foundation is crooked or crumbly, the house will never stand. Build the pose block by block on a very firm base.

Approach and Finish   Give the same careful attention to coming out of a pose as to going in. Pretend you are seeing yourself on film. Eventually you won't see any difference between running the film forward or backward.

Workout Space   You need to have a place that you can count on every day. Think of it as your Winning-Edge Workout Space. Choose a place with a firm surface and good ventilation. You don't need a lot of room. All you need is enough space to stand or lie down with your arms extended overhead and your legs and arms spread wide apart.

Whenever possible, work out in bare feet on a wood or tile floor. Use any lines on the floor to help you align your feet and legs. Square yourself to the room so that you are at right angles, perpendicular, or parallel to the floor, walls, or ceiling. Use a folded blanket or firm pad for sitting or lying poses.

Your Winning-Edge Space should be free of distractions so that you can use *all your energy* to concentrate *on yourself. You* get all your undivided attention for those so few minutes.

But don't restrict yourself to the "just right" conditions. You may never find them. *Use whatever you've got.* Recognize your ability to adjust to your environment or change it. Do whatever you can wherever you are.

Equipment   You already have the necessary equipment to practice Undercover Exercise. The nuts and bolts of *you* are all you need.

But you *can* use everything around you as your playground: furniture, ledges, walls, barrels, swings, fences, benches, doors, ties, cushions . . . whatever. The world is your playground.

Clothing You can work out in shorts and shirts, sweat clothes, leotards and tights, or any loose, comfortable clothing. Work out in bare feet. It's an elixir for your feet. If you have to wear socks, wear socks that provide good traction and lots of room for your feet.

Wear as little clothing as possible so that you can see your skin and muscles, and x-ray-view your bones more easily. Look at yourself in a mirror every once in a while. Mirrors help you to see what you're doing. But beware. You can become distracted by your image so that you miss the fun of going inside, seeing yourself with "inside eyes."

Workout Time What time of day should you work out? All day with Undercover Exercise! But the time for your Daily Winning-Edge Workout will depend on your circadian rhythm. I thrive on a morning workout and recommend it for giving that winning edge to an entire day. But some people just can't function first thing in the morning and have to do their workout later in the day or evening. Another ideal time would be immediately after work. It's lethal to plunk your tired body down and watch television. Usually, the evening ends there. Instead, flop onto the floor and do the Supine Leg Stretch. It's your shot in the arm instead of a shot in the glass.

Work out before you eat or at least one and a half hours after a meal. But don't let the excuse "I've just eaten" keep you from doing a few poses. The section Under The Tablecloth in Chapter 7 will show you what you can do before and after a meal to help digestion.

Alignment Awareness We are all asymmetrical to some degree. As you practice, you will learn very quickly about your own asym-metry. One side of your body will be dominant over the other. Work your less dominant side longer than the dominant side. Close observation of your body will make you more aware of your alignment. Misalignment causes stress, strain, and injury to the body. As you practice, create good alignment, even though you're not perfectly symmetrical. Compare the right side of your body to the left. At first you'll notice only gross differences, but as you practice you will be able to compare the differences at more subtle levels. Once you're a master at comparing your right side to your left, then you can compare yourself to other people. Most of us never live that long!

Foot and Knee Alignment

For Mountain Pose. See Figure 3.61.

- Stand with your feet hip-width apart or together.
- Pass an imaginary line through the center of your heel, sole, and second toe. The line through the right foot should be parallel to the line through the left.
- Lift your toes and spread them wide apart. Then slowly place each toe on the floor, keeping it long and in its own space. The toes are for balancing, not gripping.
- Lift one heel at a time. Stretch the sole away from your toes as you slowly lower each heel to the floor.
- Press downward on the center of each heel pad. Mountain Pose teaches you

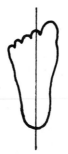 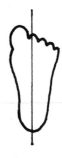

FIGURE 3.61

how to align your feet in any standing position. These principles of foot placement apply to all the standing poses.

For Standing Poses

- Start in Mountain Pose.
- For Triangle and Split-Leg Forward Bend, step your feet wide apart about the length of one leg. The distance will be wider for Lunges.
- Pivoting on the heel, turn your right foot and leg 90° to the right. Slightly flex your right knee and rotate it until your knee is in line with your second toe (Figure 3.62).

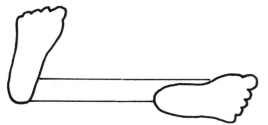
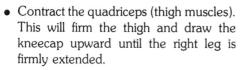

FIGURE 3.62

- Contract the quadriceps (thigh muscles). This will firm the thigh and draw the kneecap upward until the right leg is firmly extended.
- Pivoting on the heel, turn the left foot 15° inward so that it points toward the midline of your body.
- If your feet roll to the inside edges, concentrate on pressing down the outside edges. If your feet roll to the outside edges, concentrate on pressing down the inside edges. Balance!

When you are doing groin stretch poses, like Triangle and Fencer's Pose, the foot placement shown in Figure 3.62 may not accommodate tight hips and inner thigh muscles. Adjust your feet so that they line up heel to arch, as in Figure 3.63A. As you progress, you can align the feet heel to heel again. This will increase the groin stretch.

You may find it difficult to keep your balance in closed groin poses like Warrior and Split-Leg Forward Bend. If so, step your feet apart several inches. As you turn your torso, your heels will be in line with your hip joints. This allows a broader base and greater stability. See Figure 3.63B.

Make sure that the midline of your knee is in line with your second toe in everything you do. This will minimize torque to the knee and allow the muscles, tendons, and ligaments around the knee to support the joint. Pressing downward on the *center* of each heel will keep your legs strong and aligned properly.

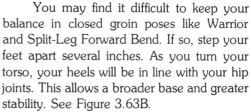
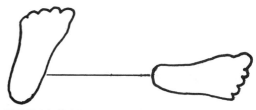

FIGURE 3.63 (a)

To check for hyperextended knees, hold a yardstick beside your leg so that it passes over your hip and ankle joints. Your knee hyperextends if it presses backward in a convex curve behind the line of the yardstick.

If your knees tend to hyperextend, slightly flex your knees. Press your shin bones forward and firm the thighs. Concentrate on relaxing the back of the knees, extending the knee joints in a Two-Way Stretch.

Relaxation At the end of all the configurations, you will be taught the Relaxation Pose. It will teach you how to let go and relax. *End your workout with a 5- to 15-minute Relaxation Pose.* This allows time for processing what you've experienced and renewal of energy.

Now let's get started with Configuration 1. Spend 5 minutes doing the One-Legger and One-Legger Twist. Notice how good you

feel after those exercises and how easy they
are to do during your day.

Configuration 1: One-Leggers

These poses lengthen hamstrings; strengthen
and shape the legs; release tension in neck,
shoulders, buttocks, and legs; develop balance and coordination; and reduce back
fatigue. One-Leggers make up one of the
most useful group of poses for everyday situations.

One-Legger (Variation of Utthita Hasta Padangusthasana)

- Stand in Mountain Pose. Apply Cosmic
  Sandwich.
- Lift one leg and place it on a stool, the
  rung of a chair, or a ledge. See Figure
  3.64.
- Stretch the back of the lifted leg.
- Keep the foot aligned with your knee
  and hip joint.
- Exhale and bend forward over the lifted
  leg. Use Fulcrum-Lever Concept.
- Go down only as far as you can maintain Cosmic Sandwich. Don't collapse in
  the waistline.
- Keep your hands clasped behind your
  back, as in Coffee Break Stretch; or
  grasp the lifted leg (Figure 3.65).

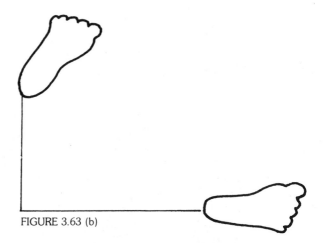

FIGURE 3.63 (b)

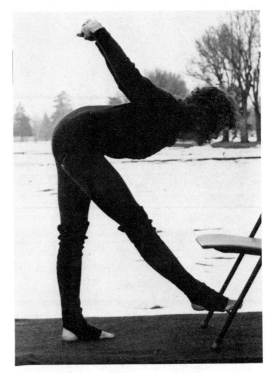

FIGURE 3.64

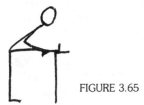

FIGURE 3.65

- Exhaling, return to an upright position.
- Repeat, lifting the other leg.
- There are many times during the day
  when you can do One-Legger without
  the forward bend; just put one leg up on
  a prop.

One-Legger Twist

- Begin in the One-Legger position with
  one leg on a chair or ledge (Figure
  3.66).
- Stretch your arms out to your sides at
  shoulder level, palms down.

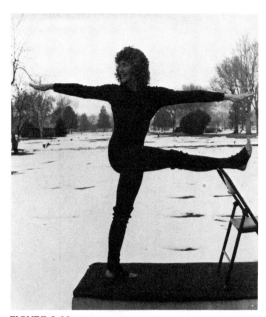

FIGURE 3.66

- Exhaling, turn your torso, head, and arms like a weather vane to the side of the lifted leg. Keep your chin parallel to the floor, and your eyes looking over your back arm.
- Stretch through your arms and turn your torso from the navel. Your legs are very straight.
- If you have a wall, ledge, or furniture around you, use it to help you turn. Brace one hand on the prop, the other on your upper leg, and move into the turn. Do not lose the alignment of your base. Maintain Cosmic Sandwich.
- Exhale, return to the starting position, and lower your arms.
- Repeat with the opposite leg, turning to the opposite side.

Flying One-Legger (Virabhadrasana III)

- Stand in Mountain Pose torso-length from a chair or ledge. Face the chair or ledge.
- Inhaling, stretch your arms out in front

of you and then up toward the ceiling. Do Cosmic Sandwich.

- On an exhalation, stand on one leg and let your arms, torso, and opposite straight leg fly out parallel to the floor over the standing leg. Rest your arms on the chair back (optional). See Figure 3.67.
- Keep your arms, torso, and lifted leg parallel to the floor and in alignment. Your standing leg is perpendicular to the floor and both hips are level.
- Exhaling, pivot back to starting position.
- Do the pose on the other leg.

Tree Pose (Vrksasana)

- Stand 3 to 4 inches away from a wall in Mountain Pose. Rest your back against the wall.
- Place your left foot against the inside of the lower right leg.
- Turn the left knee out to the side until the right hip begins to leave the wall. Stop there.
- Press both buttocks against the wall.
- Lift your left foot until you can grasp the ankle with your left hand.
- Firmly contract your right thigh muscles. Press your left foot against the inner right thigh.

FIGURE 3.67

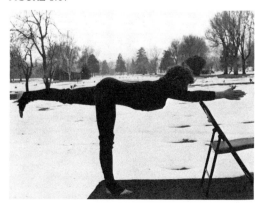

- Breathe quietly and focus on a point opposite you to help you balance.
- Now inhale and stretch the arms up over your head until your thumbs touch the wall.
- Keep your shoulders *down* as you stretch *up* with your arms in a Two-Way Stretch.
- Hold the pose, breathing quietly.
- Exhaling, lower your arms and then the leg.
- Repeat, standing on the other leg.
- Now practice Tree Pose away from the wall. See Figure 3.68.

Standing Eagle (Variation of Garudasana)

- Stand in Mountain Pose.

FIGURE 3.68

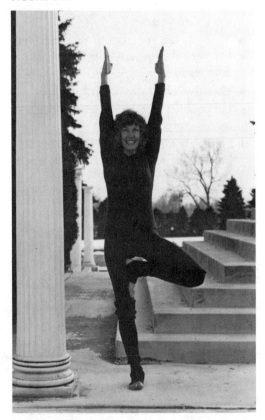

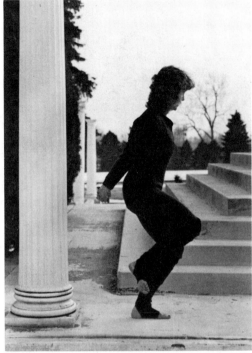

FIGURE 3.69

- Bend your left leg, keeping the foot on the floor.
- Wrap your right foot around the shin of your left leg, positioning the toes and ball of the foot beside your left foot.
- Press your left knee into the back of your right knee.
- Drop your hips as though you were going to sit on an imaginary chair.
- Clasp your hands behind you, or hold onto a prop.
- If you can keep your balance, lift your right leg and bring it across your left thigh. Hook the right foot around the left calf. (See Figure 3.69.) If your foot won't go around the calf, just press the outside of your right foot against the lower left leg.
- Feel the stretch in your hip joints and at the back of your pelvis. This is a good pose for tired legs and back.

- Exhale and return to starting position. Change legs.

Configuration 2: Angles

These poses develop balanced torso strength, lengthen hamstrings, and firm the legs. They incorporate easily into travel and office routine.

Triangle (Utthita Trikonasana)

- Stand in Mountain Pose with your right side near a wall. Place a chair to your left about 4½ feet from the wall.
- Step your feet one leg-length apart, placing the side of your right foot against the wall.
- Pivot on your left heel, turning the foot out 90° to the side. Turn your right foot inward.
- Keep your legs firmly extended throughout this pose. Lift your arches and your kneecaps.
- Stretch your arms and hands sideways at shoulder level, palms down.
- Exhaling, stretch your side out over the left leg. Grasp the back of the chair and use it to help elongate your torso as you stretch parallel to the floor.
- Exhaling, push the floor downward with your feet and legs. Feel your torso lengthen.
- Use your abdominals to support your torso in Cosmic Sandwich.
- Lower your left arm until your hand rests on your shin bone.
- Exhaling, stretch your right arm and hand up over your head. Feel as though you are reaching for the branch of a tree. See Figure 3.70.
- Keep your torso parallel to the floor, your legs supporting your torso.
- Now tuck your chin and turn your head. Look at the upper hand.

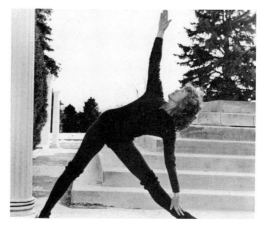

FIGURE 3.70

- Keep the back of your neck long and extended.
- Work in this position, breathing quietly.
- Exhale and, like a windmill, bring your arms and torso erect again.
- Do the Triangle to the opposite side.

Split-Leg Forward Bend (Parsvottanasana)

- Stand in Mountain Pose.
- Place your legs and feet in Triangle position to the left.
- Exhaling, stretch your arms behind you and grasp your elbows, or place hands palms together and little fingers against the spine.
- Exhaling, turn your torso to the left.

FIGURE 3.71

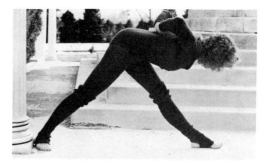

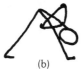

FIGURE 3.72

- Level your hips.
- Exhaling, rotate your pelvis forward. Your torso is parallel to the floor.
- Work in the pose, breathing rhythmically. Create a Two-Way Stretch from hips to crown of skull (Figure 3.71).
- Exhaling, extend outward and downward, bringing your torso closer to your thigh (Figure 3.72).
- Maintain Cosmic Sandwich. If you collapse in the middle of your torso, you've gone too far. Work in the position where you can keep the lever straight.
- Exhale and lift your torso and head to an erect position. Use your Core Power.
- Turn to the center and do the pose to the opposite side.

90° Forward Bend (Variation of Dandasana)

- Stand in Mountain Pose facing the wall.
- Place your hands on the wall at hip level.
- Walk your hips away from the wall until your torso is at a 90°-angle with your legs, forming a Suspension Bridge or 90° Forward Bend.
- Draw your shoulders away from your head. Arms are shoulder-width apart.
- Contract your thighs and watch your kneecaps pull upward as you extend your legs. Keep pressing your heels *downward* and drawing your thighs *upward* in a Two-Way Stretch.
- As you exhale, walk up the wall with your hands. "Let your fingers do the walking" until you can stand again in Mountain Pose.

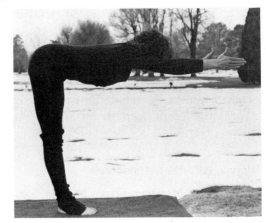

FIGURE 3.73

- Do the pose away from the wall when your back and abdominal muscles are strong enough to support your spine. (Figure 3.73.)

Dog Stretch (Adho Mukha Svanasana)

- Assume Table Pose with the top of your head touching a wall and your middle fingers touching the baseboard. If your shoulders are stiff or tight, widen the distance between your hands.
- Draw your shoulders away from your ears.
- Create and maintain Cosmic Sandwich.
- Exhaling, curl toes and straighten your legs, lifting your buttocks up and away from the wall.
- Exhaling, draw your head away from the wall. See Figure 3.74.
- Press firmly on all surfaces of your hands, especially thumbs and middle fingers.
- Keep your arms long and extended, inside elbows facing each other.
- Keep your hips high as you draw your heels toward the floor.
- Create a Two-Way Stretch between your hands and hip joints and your hip joints and heels. (See Figure 3.74.)

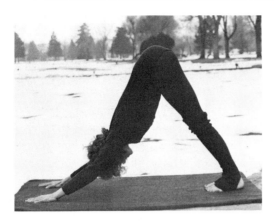

FIGURE 3.74

- Observe your knees as you work in the pose. Keep them in alignment.
- Use Dog Stretch as a warm-up or cool-down. It's a dynamic workout.

Hover Pose (Chaturanga Dandasana)

- Lie on the floor in prone position.
- Place your hands under your shoulders, fingers pointing straight ahead.
- Exhale and lift your head, torso, and legs off the floor 2 to 3 inches.
- *Hover.* Pretend you are held up by a cushion of air, balanced on your four limbs—hands and balls of feet. See Figure 3.75. If your arms can't hold your weight, drop your knees to the floor.
- Exhale and draw your body forward, parallel to the floor, as you roll onto the tops of your feet.

FIGURE 3.75

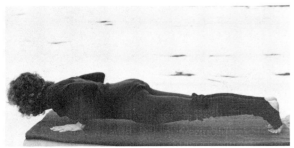

- Hover.
- Exhale, pushing backward until you're on the balls of your feet again, hands under shoulders.
- Lie on the floor and relax. (Amen!)

Configuration 3: Legs

These poses build powerful thighs, lower legs, and abdominal muscles as well as taking strain out of the lower back. They provide challenging work for the whole body and are easy to use all day long in many tasks.

Mogul (Utkatanasana)

- Stand with your hips and back against a wall.
- Exhaling, slide your hips down the wall, as in the Back Press.
- Inhaling, stretch your arms out in front of you and then up over your head. Palms face each other, thumbs toward the wall.

FIGURE 3.76

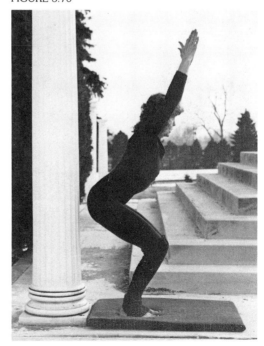

- Apply Cosmic Sandwich.
- Exhaling, rotate your pelvis forward, stretching your arms and torso out on the diagonal. See Figure 3.76.
- Notice what's happened to your Cosmic Sandwich. Adjust and realign your torso.
- Bring your arms down beside you and push off away from the wall.
- Exhaling, lift your arms above your head. Keep your torso and arms on a diagonal using Cosmic Sandwich.
- Hold the pose, breathing rhythmically.
- Exhale and stand erect.

Hot Dog

- Stand in Mountain Pose.
- Place your hands on your hips and bend both knees as much as you can, keeping both feet flat on the floor.
- Exhale and tuck your pelvis.

FIGURE 3.77

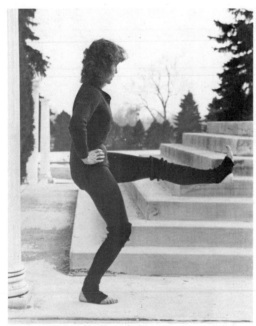

- Inhaling, extend one leg out in front of you. Place the heel on the floor.
- Stretch through the heel of the extended leg. Feel the muscles of the bent leg working.
- Exhale, and lift the extended leg.
- Dip on the bent leg and lift the extended leg as high as you can (Figure 3.77). Pretend you're moving along on one ski.
- Return to Mountain Pose and reverse legs.

Fencer's Pose (Virabhadrasana II)

- Stand with your right side next to a wall, as you did in Triangle. Step your feet one step wider apart.
- Place a chair to your left side, about 4 to 5 feet away from the wall.
- Turn your left foot 90 degrees toward the chair, your right foot slightly inward.
- Stretch your arms and hands out to the side at shoulder level, palms down.
- Exhaling, bend your left knee until it forms a 90°-angle with your lower leg and thigh.
- Keep your opposite leg firmly extended.
- Keeping your spine perpendicular to the floor, reach with your right hand for the wall and left hand for the back of the chair.
- Turn your head to look over your left arm, chin parallel to the floor.
- Breathe rhythmically. Feel as though you're pressing your legs, torso, and head between the pages of a book. Become a Cosmic Sandwich.
- Exhale, straighten the left leg, and turn your head to center.
- Change sides.
- Do Fencer's Pose without the aid of any props. (See Figure 3.78.)

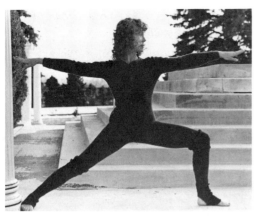

FIGURE 3.78

Runner's Lunge

- Stand in Mountain Pose.
- Place your right foot on a box or stool and stretch with your foot on a prop. See Figure 3.79.
- Exhaling, press the bent knee forward and keep the back leg firmly extended.
- Press both heels down as you breathe and stretch.
- Repeat on the other side.

FIGURE 3.79

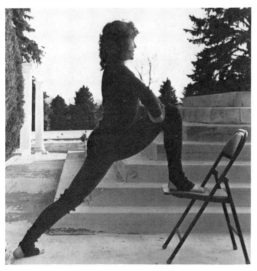

Warrior (Virabhadrasana I)

- Stand with your right side to the wall. Place your feet in Fencer's Pose starting position keeping both legs straight.
- Press your back heel against the wall and firmly extend both legs.
- Inhaling, extend your arms and hands over your head.
- Exhaling, turn your torso, arms, and head to the left.
- Level your hips and tuck your pelvis. Keep your back leg straight. If you find it difficult to turn, lift your back heel and press it to the wall.
- Exhaling, bend your left knee, forming a 90°-angle with shin and thigh bone.
- Inhaling, arch your upper thoracic spine as in Cow Pose. Stretch your arms and torso upwards.
- Lift your sternum and look upward. See Figure 3.80.

FIGURE 3.80

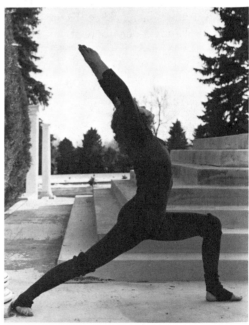

- Breathe rhythmically in the pose.
- Exhale, straighten your bent leg, and turn your torso to starting position again.
- Do Warrior to the other side.
- Repeat the exercise away from the wall. Feel the exhilaration of a proud warrior.

Configuration 4: Body Bends

These poses lengthen hamstrings, trim the waistline, massage abdominal organs, and aid digestion. They are quieting, rejuvenating poses.

Seated Forward Bend
(Paschimottanasana)

- Sit in a straight-backed chair.
- Rest your feet flat on the floor. Place a pad under your feet if they can't rest on the floor.
- Inhale, extend your arms and grasp your elbows above your head, and stretch upward from the hips.
- Exhale and tip your pelvis and spine forward, stretching your torso and arms outward in a diagonal line (Figure 3.81). Use Fulcrum-Lever Concept.

FIGURE 3.81

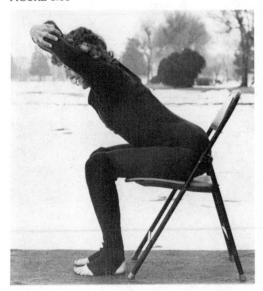

- Scoot your sitting bones toward the back of the chair.
- Separate your legs wide apart. Bring your torso, head, and arms down between your legs. Relax and hang like a rag doll for a few moments (Figure 3.82).

FIGURE 3.82

- Then, exhaling, grasp your elbows and lift your arms, head, and torso parallel to the floor.
- As you exhale, use Core Power to lift you to an erect position.
- CAUTION: If lifting your torso in this position strains your back, roll up like a rag doll to an erect position.
- Now do Seated Forward Bend sitting on the floor with a folded pad under your hips and a tie around your feet (Figure 3.83A–B).
- Exhaling, tip your pelvis-spine forward to a 45° position.
- If you can't keep your torso and legs straight, you've gone too far. Work in the position where you can maintain Cosmic Sandwich.
- Eventually you can drop the tie and grasp your calves or feet.
- Breathe quietly in the pose, lengthening and elongating your legs and spine.
- This pose is extremely beneficial when done correctly. It has been given bad reviews in recent years because it is usually done incorrectly, contributing to, rather than correcting, back problems. Cosmic Sandwich makes it possible to do this pose safely, supporting and strengthening the back.

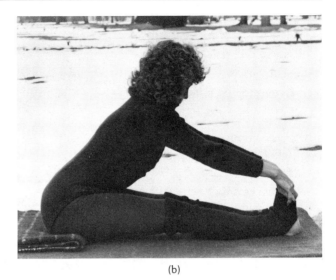

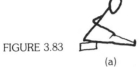

FIGURE 3.83

(a)   (b)

Sitting Leg Stretch (Janu Sirsasana)

- Sit on the floor in Staff Pose. Use a pad under your sitting bones if you need to.
- Inhale and bend your right knee, drawing the foot toward your groin.
- Exhale; turn your knee outward from the hip joint and rest it on the floor.
- Draw the right heel close to your pubic bone. Make sure the right hip is not drawn back behind the left.
- Firmly extend your left leg. Place a tie around the ball of your left foot.
- Hold onto the tie with both hands and flex your foot. Keep your arms close to your sides. See Figure 3.84.
- Exhaling, rotate your spine and pelvis forward in a diagonal line.
- Keep your chin at right angles to your throat.
- Draw the top of your head and sternum *forward* and your tailbone *backward*, creating a Two-Way Stretch.
- Breathe rhythmically and *give your hamstrings time to lengthen.*
- As the hamstrings lengthen, walk your hands along the tie toward your left foot,

drawing your torso toward your legs. Maintain Cosmic Sandwich.
- To increase the difficulty, drop the tie and place your hands around your left knee, calf, or foot.
- Rotate your pelvis farther forward until your torso rests on your left leg. Keep Cosmic Sandwich.
- Stay in the pose, breathe quietly.
- Exhale and return the pelvis-spine to an erect position.
- Repeat on the opposite side.
- Sitting Leg Stretch is a peaceful and

FIGURE 3.84

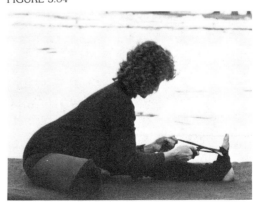

quiet pose. Don't struggle in it. Keep your alignment and Cosmic Sandwich as you practice the pose.

Supine Jackknife (Urdhva Mukha Paschimottanasana)

- Lie down on your back in alignment.
- Exhaling, draw both knees to your chest.
- Place a tie or belt across the balls of your feet (Figure 3.85).

FIGURE 3.85

- Very slowly extend your legs, hold, and relax. Repeat this procedure several times. Those of you with back or sciatic problems can practice this often until your condition improves.
- Straighten both legs. Press the inside of your heels upward, lengthening the inside of your legs.
- To increase the difficulty, slowly lower your legs toward your head to a 45° angle as you exhale (Figure 3.86). Visualize scissor blades closing.

FIGURE 3.86

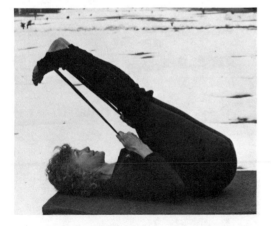

- Release the tie. Reach between your knees and grasp your big toes with your index fingers.
- Breathe rhythmically and relax in the pose. Keep your sacrum pressed to the floor.
- Release your toes and bring your legs back to the floor.

Intense Forward Bend (Uttanasana)

- Stand in Mountain Pose 12 to 15 inches away from a wall.
- Place your back and hips against the wall.
- With your hands on your hip joints, do a 90° Forward Bend.
- Exhale and stretch your torso out and downward until your hips "get stuck" on the wall. Your pelvis is tipped as much as possible.
- Don't fold in the middle. Keep the lever straight. Do Cosmic Sandwich.
- Bend your knees and press your ribs to your thighs.
- Extend your arms and place hands, palms down, on the floor beside your feet.
- If you can't touch the floor, place each hand on a pile of books.
- Gradually begin to straighten your legs, allowing time for your hamstrings to lengthen.
- Breathe quietly and hold the pose, head and face relaxed, legs and torso maintaining a Two-Way Stretch (Figure 3.87).
- Bring your hands back to your hip joints. Exhaling, use Core Power to help extend your torso back to the wall.
- Eventually you can do the pose away from the wall.
- Start with Seated Forward Bend. Work slowly and carefully, applying Tip and

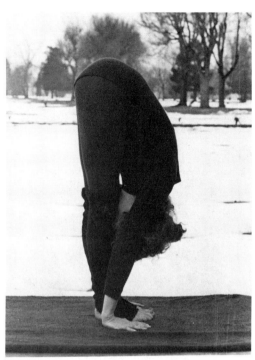

FIGURE 3.87

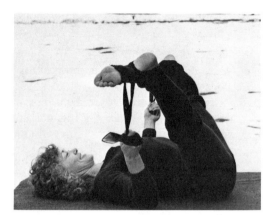

FIGURE 3.88

Tuck and Cosmic Sandwich—safe back principles for any forward bending—to strengthen your back.

Configuration 5: Spread Eagle

These poses stretch groin and hamstring muscles, permitting increased pelvic mobility. They also strengthen back and abdominal muscles.

Supine Eagle (Variation of Urdhva Mukha Paschimottanasana)

- Lie on your back in alignment.
- Bring both knees to your chest.
- Wrap a separate tie around the ball of each foot, and grasp the ends of a tie in each hand. Keep upper arms and elbows beside you.
- Exhale and stretch your legs upward.
- Exhaling, stretch the legs wide apart, keeping your back and pelvis firmly pressed to the floor (Figure 3.88).

- Breathe quietly, working in the pose.
- To increase the difficulty, bring both knees to your chest and drop your ties.
- Reach between your knees and grasp your big toes with your index fingers and thumbs.
- Exhaling, extend your legs upward and then separate them wide apart.
- Keep your back and pelvis firmly pressed to the floor.
- Feel the stretch in your arms, shoulders, and legs.
- Exhaling, bend your knees and squeeze them to your chest.
- Extend your legs on the floor and relax.

Sitting Eagle (Upavistha Konasana)

- Sit in Staff Pose on the floor. Use a pad under your sitting bones.
- Apply all the principles of Cosmic Sandwich and back safety you have learned and practiced in the Body Bends Configurations.
- Place a tie around each foot and grasp the ends of the ties (Figure 3.89).

FIGURE 3.89

- Exhaling, separate your legs as wide apart as you can.
- Keep your back very straight.
- Flex your feet and straighten your knees. If it's a struggle for you to keep both your back and legs straight, practice this pose with your back against a wall.
- To increase the difficulty, grasp your big toes. Breathe quietly and hold.
- Now grasp the inner edges of your feet (Figure 3.90). Stretch arms and legs, bringing your torso as close to the floor as you can. Keep back straight.
- Rest your forehead on the floor or cushion. Breathe quietly.
- Exhaling, draw your torso erect again, using Core Power.

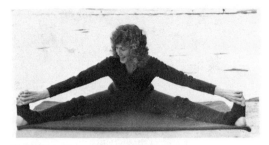

FIGURE 3.90

Eagle Balance (Variation of Ubhaya Padangusthasana)

- Sit in Staff Pose.
- Bring your knees to your chest. Reach between your knees and grasp your big toes.
- Exhaling, lift your feet off the floor and *balance* on your hips. Keep Cosmic Sandwich.
- Breathe quietly in the pose.
- Exhale and extend both legs up and out on a diagonal. Straighten your legs. (Figure 3.91). This takes a little practice (for some of us a lot!). If you roll backward, have fun rolling!
- Bring your knees to your chest again and balance.
- Return to Staff Pose.

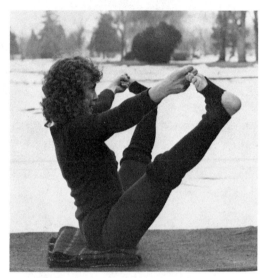

FIGURE 3.91

Bound Angle (Baddha Konasana)

- Sit on the floor in Staff Pose.
- Bring your knees to your chest.
- Now turn your knees outward, bringing the soles of your feet together, outer edges of your feet on the floor.
- Grasp your feet or ankles.
- Keep your back very straight, arms extended (Figure 3.92). If grasping your feet makes your back round, place a tie around your feet and hold onto it. Keep your arms straight.
- Exhale, and press your knees toward the floor. If you have tight groin muscles, use cushions for support under your knees.
- Keep your torso extended, sternum *up* and tailbone *down* in a Two-Way Stretch. You can practice Bound Angle against a wall, supporting your back so

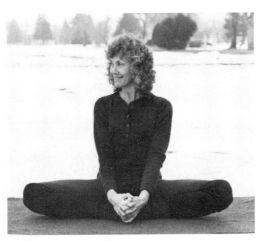

FIGURE 3.92

that you can focus more on working your legs.

- To increase the difficulty, rotate your pelvis-spine forward as you stretch your torso out over your feet (Figure 3.93).

FIGURE 3.93

- Breathe quietly. Give your groin muscles time to stretch.
- Exhale your torso erect, keeping Cosmic Sandwich.

Spread Eagle Forward Bend (Prasarita Padottanasana)

- Stand in Mountain Pose about 3 feet away from a ledge or chair.
- Step or jump your legs wide apart. Point toes straight ahead.
- Inhaling, stretch your arms overhead, palms facing in.
- Exhaling, rotate your pelvis-spine forward 90 degrees.
- Grasp the ledge or chair and create a good Two-Way Stretch.

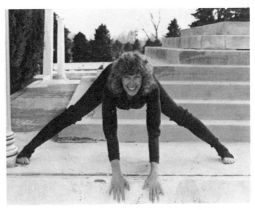

FIGURE 3.94

- Keep your legs firmly extended.
- Breathe rhythmically, giving yourself a chance to lengthen in the pose.
- Let go of the prop and exhale downward, pressing your hands to the floor, as in Dog Stretch (Figure 3.94).
- Separate your legs wide apart by walking the heels of your feet outward. Toes point inward for a better groin stretch.
- If your back rounds, you've gone too far. Use a stool or a pile of books under your hands. Elongate your spine.
- Exhale, and come up to an erect position. Use Core Power.

Configuration 6: Torso Twists

These poses increase the blood supply to tired, cramped shoulders and back, and massage the abdominals. They make you alert and responsive and are a great cure for the blahs!

Supine Torso Twist (Variation of Jathara Parivartanasana)

- Easy Back Twist is the foundation for this configuration. Go back to Back Trainers and review the pose.
- Lie on your back in alignment.
- Exhaling, bring both knees to your chest.

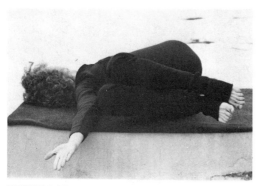

FIGURE 3.95

- Extend your arms and hands on the floor at shoulder level in *T* position. Stretch them wide apart, turning the palms up.
- Exhale, and draw your knees toward your right elbow. Bring them to the floor or let them hover several inches above the floor.
- Turn your head to the left, looking down your left arm. See Figure 3.95.
- Breathe rhythmically as you stretch your ribs, spinal column, arms, shoulders, and neck.
- Exhaling, bring your knees and torso back to center.
- Exhale and repeat to the left.
- Now extend your legs out on the floor. Exhale and lift the left leg perpendicular to the floor.
- Keep your thighs firm and both legs very straight.

- Exhale, and draw the left leg across to the right side of your body as the right leg and hip roll to the side (Figure 3.96).
- Turn your head to the left as your leg and hip turn to the right.
- Extend the left leg toward your right hand without disturbing the alignment of your shoulders, arms, or right leg.
- Hold the pose, breathing rhythmically until you're ready to come out of it.
- Exhale and return to center.
- Exhale and lower the left leg. Align yourself again.
- Exhaling, raise the right leg perpendicular to the floor. Repeat the twist to the opposite side.

Roofer's Twist (Bharadvajasana)

- Sit in Staff Pose on the floor.
- Bend both knees, and swing your feet around to the left side.
- Place your right toes over the left ankle, or keep your feet side by side.
- Grasp the right knee with your left hand.
- Press your right palm on the floor beside your right hip joint.
- Exhaling, turn your torso to the right. Keep your shoulders level. Your left hip can move forward as you turn.
- Turn from your naval using Core Power!
- Tuck your pelvis and make the spine elongate as you turn.
- Look over your left shoulder and then

FIGURE 3.96

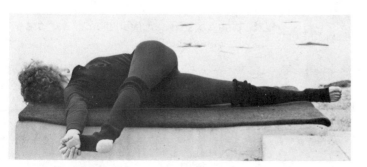

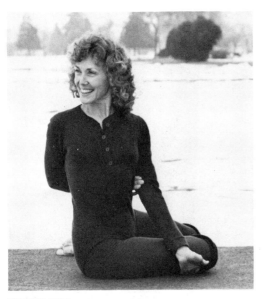

FIGURE 3.97

your right. Rotate your head slowly, keeping your chin parallel to the floor.

- Stretch your right arm around your back and grasp your left arm. To increase the difficulty, slide your left hand, palm down, under your knee (Figure 3.97).
- Hold the twist and breathe rhythmically until you are ready to come out of the pose.
- Exhale and turn to center.
- Bring your legs to center, swing them around to the opposite side, and repeat the twist.
- This pose is named for the workers who kneel and twist to lay a new roof.

Sitting Twists *(Marichyasana III)*

- Sit in Staff Pose with your right side 6 inches from a wall. Place a pad under your sitting bones if you need one.
- Now bend your right knee and draw your heel close to your right hip joint.
- Extend your left leg firmly.

- Grasp your right knee with your left hand.
- Press your right hand to the wall and turn toward the wall.
- When you've turned as far as you can, keeping your hips and shoulders level, place your right hand beside your right hip joint and continue turning to the right.
- If you have twisted as far as you can, release the right knee and use your left elbow like a rudder against your outer right knee. Press the left hand to the wall (Figure 3.98).
- Squeeze your thighs together.
- Keep your shoulders level.
- Rotate your head toward the right and then slowly to the left, keeping your chin at right angles to your throat.
- Hold, breathing rhythmically, until you're ready to come out of the pose.
- Exhale and release the stretch, turning back to center.
- Turn your left side to the wall and repeat the twist.
- If this pose is difficult, do another variation of it: Use the same starting position, but bend the leg farthest from the wall instead of closest to it. Follow the same procedure for twisting.

FIGURE 3.98

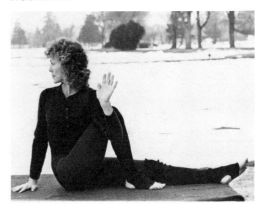

Configuration 7: Bow

Great energizers, Bow poses lengthen hip flexors and quadriceps; strengthen hamstring, buttock, back, and core muscles for a balanced backbend; and they expand the chest and work out arm and shoulder tension.

Standing Bow (Variation of Natarajasana)

- Stand in Mountain Pose facing a wall, with your feet about six inches away from the wall.
- Place your right hand on the wall at shoulder level.
- Stand on your right leg. Bend your left knee and bring the heel toward your hip. Grasp the left ankle with your left hand. Use a tie if you need to.
- Tuck your pelvis and press your pubic bone toward the wall. Maintain this Tuck position.
- Point your left knee gradually downward until your thighs and knees are parallel to each other. If this causes compression in your lower back, keep your knee pointing toward the wall. Keep your shoulders and hips parallel to the floor.
- Stretch your right arm up the wall as far as you can. If possible grasp a ledge to help you stretch.
- Inhaling, arch your thoracic spine upward as in Cow Pose. Keep your pelvis tucked. Use Dynamic Duo. See Figure 3.99.
- Slowly release your leg and come back into Mountain Pose. Repeat on the other side.

Ballet Bow

- Assume Standing Bow about 2 to 3 feet from a table or ledge.
- Draw your bent knee back behind you until you cannot keep your pelvis tucked.

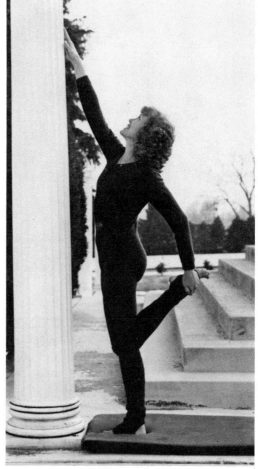

FIGURE 3.99

- Then rotate your pelvis-spine forward over the fulcrum-hip joint of the standing leg.
- Reach for the ledge. Level your shoulders and hips as you hold your torso and bent leg parallel to the floor. See Figure 3.100.
- Breathe rhythmically as you work in the pose.
- To vary the pose, change your grasp from the outside to the inside of your ankle. Turn your torso to the side and stretch (Figure 3.101).
- Keep your standing leg firmly extended.

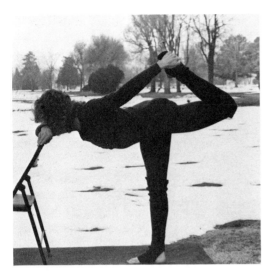

FIGURE 3.100

- Turn your head to look at your lifted leg.
- Point the knee downward, not sideways. Exhaling, draw your foot back behind you. Feel as though you're drawing an arrow on the string of a bow.

- When you're ready to come out of the pose, exhale and lower the leg. Turn your body forward.
- Return to Mountain Pose and do Ballet Bow on the opposite side.

One-Step Backbend

- Cobra Pose and Coffee Break Stretch are preparation for all backbending. Go back to Back Trainers and review these first.
- Stand in Mouutain Pose, your back about 2 to 3 inches away from the wall.
- Step one foot forward, firming your base.
- Inhaling, extend your arms up over head.
- Exhaling, lace your fingers together and press palms *upward* and heels *downward* in a Two-Way Stretch.
- Release your fingers and turn them to touch the wall, palms up. Keep arms ex-

FIGURE 3.101

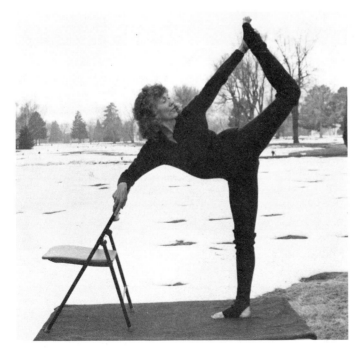

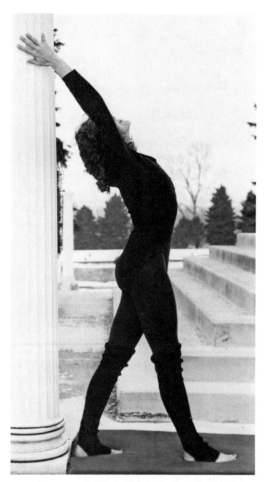

FIGURE 3.102

Upward Dog Stretch (Urdhva Mukha Svanasana)

- Lie on the floor in prone position as in Cobra Pose, forehead down.
- Place your feet hip-width apart and your hands beside your chest, palms down.
- Exhaling, tuck your pelvis. Use Dynamic Duo. Maintain the tuck throughout the pose.
- Exhale and pull your chest forward and upward as you straighten your arms.
- Lift your torso and thighs off the floor, while keeping your lower legs and feet on the floor.
- Look straight ahead, chin parallel to the floor.
- If you can maintain Dynamic Duo, lift your knees and lower legs off the floor. Your hands and feet are now the base. (See Figure 3.103.)
- Inhaling, draw your chest upward through your arms, like thread passing through a needle. Stay on your toes as in Figure 3.103 or let your feet flip, soles facing upward.
- Just let your head follow the direction of the movement.
- Draw your shoulders down away from your ears. Feel light and strong. Notice your breathing quicken as you work in the pose.

FIGURE 3.103

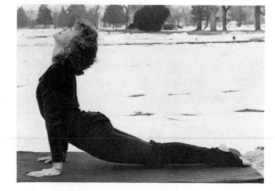

tended. Do the pose where you can grasp a door jamb or ledge if necessary. See Figure 3.102.

- Inhale and lift your sternum upward, arching your thoracic spine as you tuck your pelvis.
- Shift your weight to the forward leg as you lift your back heel. Push off from the ball of your back foot. Turn on Core Power!
- Exhaling, step forward with the back foot, and rise up on your toes. Then stand in Mountain Pose.
- Repeat with the opposite leg forward.

- Exhaling, bend your elbows and slowly return to the floor. Relax.
- Use Dynamic Duo for all backbending. Use this sophisticated and polished system of balanced muscle action to elongate your spine from tailbone to base of skull.

Configuration 8: Bottoms Up

These poses build shoulder, arm, wrist, and hand strength; develop core muscle strength, balance, and harmony; and reverse the pull of gravity on the body and increase the blood supply to the brain. (Avoid during menstruation.)

Handstand (Adho Mukha Vrksasana)

- Assume Table Pose with your backside to the wall, the soles of your feet touching the wall.
- Exhale into Dog Stretch. Press your heels to the wall and your toes and the balls of your feet to the floor.
- Bend your right knee. Press the foot to the wall about 1 or 2 feet above the floor.
- Push off with your right foot against the wall.
- Exhale as you lift your left leg to the wall.
- Walk your feet up the wall. See Figure 3.104.
- Keep your shoulders wide apart and away from your ears.
- Undergird your back with powerful Core Power!
- Extend your body up the wall on a diagonal. *Breathe!* This can be scary at first, especially if you've never done it before. Have someone stand beside you to "spot" or support you if you need it.
- When you're brave enough to try another version of Handstand, turn around and do Dog Stretch with your head toward the wall and with your hands about 1 foot away from the wall.

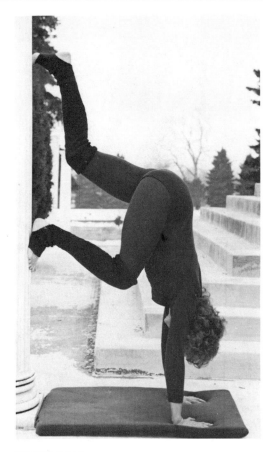

FIGURE 3.104

- Bending the right knee, step forward with the right foot.
- Lift your head slightly as you look between your hands.
- Exhaling, push off with the right leg and pull upward with the left toward the ceiling.
- Use your airlift to swing up lightly against the wall, feet resting on the wall. You can have someone stand beside you and guide your legs, but don't let anyone else lift them for you.
- Turn on Core Power and tuck your pelvis.
- Stretch toward the ceiling with the inside of your feet and legs.

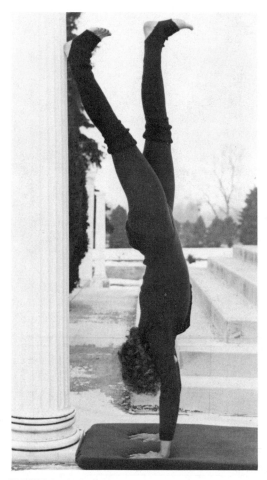

FIGURE 3.105

- Feel each finger and palm as you work your hands to balance.
- Continue practicing with your feet against the wall and then away from the wall until you can stand free. See Figure 3.105.
- When you're ready to come down, lower your legs one at a time.

Half Headstand (Variation of Salamba Sirsasana)

- Assume Table Pose with your hands several inches from a wall.
- Place your forearms on the floor.

- Cup your hands around your elbows. This forms one line of the equilateral triangle that will become your base.
- Release the elbows and lace your fingers together without moving the position of your elbows. The three lines—knuckles to elbows and elbow to elbow—form the triangle.
- Place the crown of your head to the floor between your hands and arms.
- Rest the back of your skull against your palms (Figure 3.106).

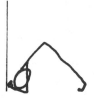

FIGURE 3.106

- Press down firmly on elbows and wrists.
- Lift your shoulders *upward* and press your elbows *downward* in a Two-Way Stretch.
- The head may lightly touch the floor or clear it by "a hair." Let the head hang in traction. Feel the elongation at the back of your neck.
- Keep your chin parallel to the floor.
- Exhaling, straighten your legs and lift your hips upward, keeping your feet on the floor.
- Breathe rhythmically as you work your legs and create Cosmic Sandwich.
- Build strength in your base by pushing downward with your forearms and side of hands, keeping pressure off the head and neck.
- Now draw your head and torso away from your hands, letting your head hang between your arms. Stretch from elbows to hips. (See Figure 3.107).
- Inhale, and move your head and torso back to your thumbs, keeping your legs straight.

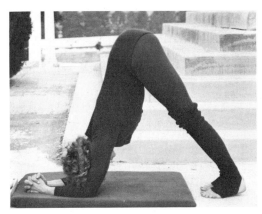

FIGURE 3.107

- Repeat this as many times as your ability and strength permit.
- Bring your knees to the floor and relax in Child's Pose.

Half Shoulderstand (Variation of Salamba Sarvangasana)

- Desk Pose forms the foundation for Half Shoulderstand. Review it in Back Trainers before practicing this pose.
- Lie down on your side with both feet to the wall, knees bent and legs forming a right angle. Hips and knees are equidistant from the wall.
- Place the pad you used for Desk Pose at your back. Arrange it so that you can roll onto it. The upper edge should extend 2 inches above your shoulders; the lower edge should be under your waistline.
- Roll your back onto the pad.
- Place your feet on the wall, legs forming a 90° angle. You are in the starting position of Desk Pose except your feet are on the wall.
- Exhale, press your feet to the wall and airlift your tucked pelvis 1 foot off the floor. Keep tucking your pelvis and keep your lumbar spine elongated, just as you did in Desk Pose.

- Hold in this position breathing rhythmically. *Visualize your hips held up by a sling.*
- Keeping your elbows as close together as you can, place your hands under your hips. This reminds me of a butler serving the Christmas ham!
- Exhaling, bring one leg away from the wall extending it on a diagonal line over your torso.
- Support the weight of your hips and legs over your hands and arms, not your shoulders.
- Bring the opposite leg parallel to the first.
- Balance the weight of your legs and pelvis on your arms, elbows, and hands. Your legs and torso form a 90° angle, as in Staff Pose. You are a Cosmic Sandwich. See Figure 3.108.
- Breathe quietly, enjoying the tranquility of the pose.
- To come out of the pose, bend your

FIGURE 3.108

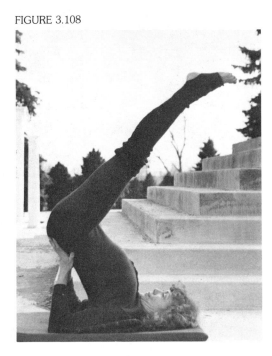

knees and bring your feet back to the wall.

- Stretch your arms behind your head and lower your spine one vertebra at a time. Let your neck arch, tipping chin upward as you come down.

Configuration 9: Bar Hang

These poses develop arm, chest, shoulders, and core strength. They put your spine in traction, your mind in action.

Bar Hang

- Stand in Mountain Pose under a chin-up bar or hanging bar. Make sure it is secure and can bear your weight.

- Grasp the bar, hands shoulder-width or more apart.

- Hang there, breathing quietly and stretching your back. Let your legs hang or rest on the floor.

- Exhaling, bring one or both knees toward your chest in a Single or Double Knee Lift. See Figure 3.109A.

- Inhale and exhale as you hold.

- To increase the abdominal work, exhale and lift and extend one or both legs. Hold them parallel to the floor in a Single or Double Leg Lift. See Figure 3.109B−C.

- In Undercover Exercise you will often

FIGURE 3.109

(a)

(b)

(c)

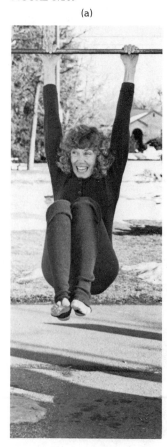
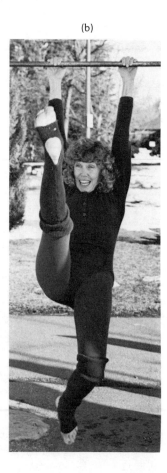
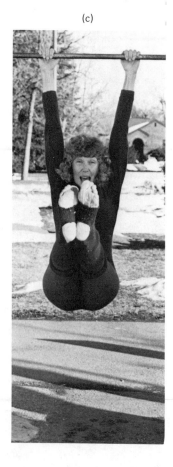

use the Single or Double Knee and Leg Lifts while sitting in a chair.

Hanging Bow (Variation of Dhanurasana)

- Have someone help you the first few times you practice this pose.
- Place a chair under an exercise bar.
- Hold onto the bar with your hands wider than shoulder-width apart.
- Exhaling, swing your legs up between your arms and hook your knees over the bar. Your legs will be like clips holding you to the bar.
- Have your partner support you as you let go with your hands and hang. Reach for the chair. See Figure 3.110.
- Tuck your pelvis and let gravity pull your spine in a Two-Way Stretch.
- Swing free of the chair and hang for a few rhythmical breaths.
- Exhaling, arch upward and grasp each ankle, one at a time (See Figure 7.23, page 153).
- Inhaling, expand your chest. Keep your pelvis tucked. You're in Hanging Bow. Mazel Tov! You did it.
- When you're ready to come out of the pose, return your hands to the bar and lower your legs one at a time.

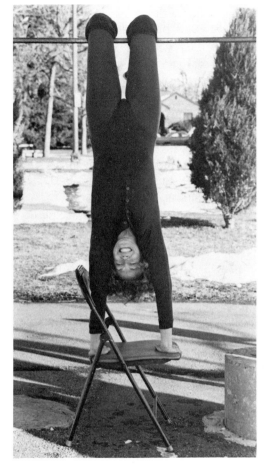

FIGURE 3.110

Configuration 10: Sun Power

Here's a grand salute to sun energy! This series of poses linked by the breath develops body strength, stamina, and endurance, and can be an aerobic workout. All poses are taken from the other configurations.

Sun Swings (Surya Namaskar)

- Stand in Mountain Pose.
- Place your hands in Namaste position. Namaste is a greeting in Sanskrit meaning, "That which in me is also in you, greets you." For Namaste position, place your palms together in prayer position, thumbs against sternum, fingers pointing outward (Figure 3.111A). Keep all surfaces of palms and fingers touching except the well of space in the center of your palms.
- Draw the elbows backward without separating your hands. This stretches the upper chest and shoulder muscles.
- Exhale, and sweep your arms in an arc downward and out to your sides.
- Inhale, and without breaking the rhythm, bring your extended arms and hands up over your head (Figure 3.111B). Arms and hands are

shoulder-width apart, palms facing inward and thumbs pointing backward.

- Lift your sternum, and lengthen your torso. Keep your head balanced between your arms, gaze upward or straight ahead.
- Exhale into Intense Forward Bend using 90° Forward Bend position as you go down. (Figure 3.111C). Inhale.
- Exhale, stepping your right leg back into Runner's Lunge (Figure 3.111D) and then inhale.
- Exhale into Dog Stretch, stepping your left leg back to meet the right (Figure 3.111E).
- Inhale, and swing into Upward Dog Stretch (Figure 3.111F). Keep your legs very straight.
- Exhale, and swing into Dog Stretch (Figure 3.111G). Inhale.
- Exhale, and step the right leg forward between your knees in Runner's Lunge (Figure 3.111H).
- Inhale and lift the hips, bringing the back leg forward into Intense Forward Bend (Figure 3.111I).

- Exhale and stretch upward with arms extended in front of you as in 90° Forward Bend. (For bad backs, stretch arms out to your side or behind you as in Coffee Break Stretch) (Figure 3.111J).
- Inhale stretching your arms and torso upward and slightly backward using Dynamic Duo (Figure 3.111K).
- Exhale, and repeat the next cycle, stepping your left leg backward and forward.
- You have just completed one *set:* one cycle stepping the right leg backward and forward and the next cycle stepping the left leg backward and forward. A cycle is one-half of a set. At the end of the set, exhale and bring your hands back to Namaste position. Stand in Mountain Pose.
- Listen to the sound of your breathing and monitor the rhythm of your heart beat. Take a moment to experience the incredible energy within and around you.
- Practice each pose in the Sun Swing very slowly at first. Breathe rhythmically for three or four breaths in each posi-

FIGURE 3.111

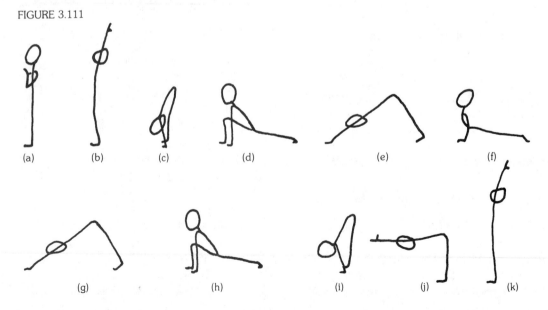

(a)   (b)   (c)   (d)   (e)   (f)

(g)   (h)   (i)   (j)   (k)

tion. Take time to observe your alignment and make any adjustments.

- Then practice the Sun Swing using the breathing pattern in the directions and on the chart.

- To build upper body and leg strength, add more swings per cycle. It's fun! Swing back and forth from Upward to Downward Dog Stretch, keeping your legs strong and springy. Let your body breathe you! Do two or three extra swings per cycle. Work up to as many as you can do. This is a grand aerobic strengthener when combined nonstop with the rest of the Sun Swing.

When you are strong enough to do the Sun Swings aerobically, you can change the breathing to suit yourself. I use an alternate pattern shown below the Breathing Pattern Chart, Breathing System II.

Breathing Pattern for Sun Swings

exhale	Mountain Pose	inhale
exhale	Intense Forward Bend	inhale
exhale	Runner's Lunge	inhale
exhale	Dog Stretch	
inhale	Upward Dog Stretch	
exhale	Dog Stretch	inhale
exhale	Runner's Lunge	
inhale	Intense Forward Bend	
exhale	Mountain Pose	inhale
	Repeat	

Breathing System II for Sun Swings When you do these aerobically, try changing the pattern so that you inhale into Runner's Lunge, exhale into Dog Stretch, inhale into Upward Dog Stretch, exhale again into Dog Stretch, inhale into Runner's Lunge, exhale into Intense Forward Bend, and inhale into Mountain Pose. Then exhale and repeat another cycle.

Jumping Sun (Surya Namaskar)

- Stand in Mountain Pose
- Inhale, and swing your arms up toward the ceiling, either out to the side and up or straight forward and up. (Figure 3.112A.)
- Exhale into 90° Forward Bend and then down into Intense Forward Bend. (Figure 3.112B.)
- Inhale, stretching your chest and head forward.
- Exhale, and jump both feet back into Hover Pose (Figure 3.112C. See also Figure 3.75.)
- Hover.
- Inhale, drawing your body forward onto the tops of your feet, and stretch upward into Upward Dog Stretch. (Figure 3.112D.)
- Exhale back into Hover Pose. (Figure 3.112E.)
- Hover. Inhale.
- Exhale, and push up and back, lifting your body into Dog Stretch. (Figure 3.112F.)
- Inhale, lifting your hips upward; bend your knees and jump both feet forward between your hands into Intense Forward Bend. (Figure 3.112G.)
- Exhale and extend into Mountain Pose stretching your arms upward. (Figure 3.112H.)
- Inhale, and repeat the cycle.

Breathing Pattern for Jumping Sun

exhale	Mountain Pose	inhale
exhale	Intense Forward Bend	inhale
exhale	Hover Pose	
inhale	Upward Dog Stretch	
exhale	Hover Pose	inhale
exhale	Dog Stretch	
inhale	Intense Forward Bend	
exhale	Mountain Pose	inhale

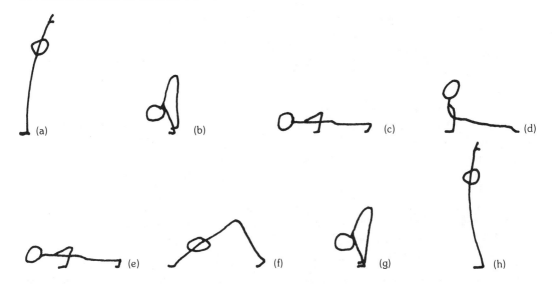

FIGURE 3.112

AEROBIC WORKOUT

Apply your training in body alignment and spinal extension to running, walking, swimming, bicycling, rowing, skiing, skating, aerobic exercise, and dancing. You'll eliminate a host of injuries as you increase your efficiency, and do so with grace and style.

Some people have to make extreme adaptations in order to get around at all. Look at the ingenuity Buford Harris has shown in getting his aerobic workout (Figure 3.113). He has the grit and determination to do the best he can with the best that he has. Some of us need to make adaptations too in order to get a good workout. I've had to make a few myself. I really enjoyed running and thought I'd run until I was 135. Luckily, I had some other passions—yoga, biking, skiing, swimming, and good old fashioned walking—because after three years of running, I had to stop. My joints just couldn't handle it. I rediscovered Sun Power and experimented with making it an aerobic substitute for running . . . a *symphony* of beautiful movements set to the harmony and rhythm of breathing.

When you try it the first time, you may not like it. It's not as easy as walking or running. It seems complicated at first and it's hard to remember what comes next. It's easy to miss the rhythm and music when you're struggling with the pose. That's what happened to me when I first tried it. I felt clumsy, and no one likes to feel clumsy! But I saw the potential for a dynamic workout, so I kept at it. Now it's my survival kit.

You can survive on it . . . and thrive on it. All you need is a space approximately 7 by 5 feet and 7 feet high. No special equipment, no special clothing. That doesn't make Sun Power very marketable for sports equipment and clothing industries, but for you, the consumer, it's a bargain!

Look at what you get: a release of tension; youthful look and carriage; spirit; full range of motion in all your joints; strong, stable, and supple spine; an alert, clear, uncluttered mind; and aerobic conditioning. My word! There must be a way to market all that! But the best things in life are still free, and this is one of them. Here's how you make it aerobic.

Practice Sun Swings or Jumping Sun, slowly at first, as described in Configuration

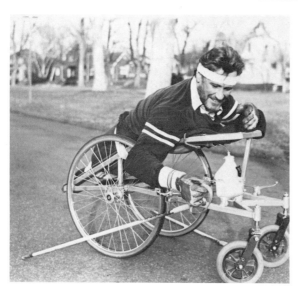
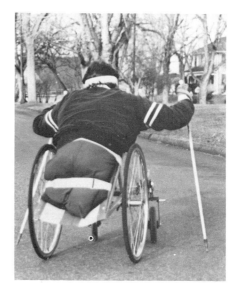

FIGURE 3.113

10: Sun Power. When you are comfortable with your form and alignment, you are ready to increase your speed and number of cycles . . . gradually please!

KEY IDEA: For cardiovascular strengthening, move quickly and steadily without pausing, accelerating your heart rate for 20 to 30 minutes four times a week. Get your doctor's approval. For the training effect, increase your work load by increasing the speed and number of cycles. When you really get going aerobically, you'll be breathing any way you can. You'll be wet with sweat and breathing through your mouth as when you run.

I have used Dr. Kenneth Cooper's formulas for getting my target heart rate and adapting Sun Power as an aerobic exercise. If you are interested in checking out the aerobic training potential for yourself, use his formulas outlined in *The Aerobics Program for Total Well-Being,* on pages 125–130. See if you have the stamina for even five minutes of Sun Swings and/or Jumping Suns at your own target heart rate. It takes quite a bit of patient training to be able to do this for 20 to 30 minutes. You will see that the upper body strength you are building in Sun Power is

considerable, to say nothing of the leg strength! It takes time for your muscles to be able to accommodate that work. Start for one minute going all out, increase gradually to five minutes, and build strength and aerobic capacity until you can sustain 20 to 30 minutes of target heart rate exercise in Sun Power. If you can't do Sun Power at target heart rate, don't let that stop you. Do it anyway! Your heart rate *will* accelerate. Keep going as long as you can. You will improve your strength, coordination, circulation, and total physical condition. It's fun, and well worth your effort!

Trouble Spots in Sun Swings

Q: Why does my leg get stuck when I bring it forward from Dog Stretch to Runner's Lunge?

A: Swing your *whole body forward,* not just your leg. Push off with your back foot. Make room for the bent leg by pushing off on your fingertips. Bring the bent leg forward with the momentum of your body.

Q: My wrists and arms are so weak. How can I get them strong enough for Upward Dog Stretch?

A: Lift weights, join Nautilus, and squeeze rubber balls all day! Or, just do it! Your wrists and arms will strengthen by doing the task. Here's a way to help yourself. From Dog Stretch, lower your knees as in Table Pose. Bend your elbows slightly as you inhale into Upward Dog Stretch. Don't hunch your shoulders. Create Dynamic Duo.

Q: Will I ever be able to straighten my legs?

A: Hamstrings increase in length with consistent, persistent stretching, but lengthening enough to allow you to fully straighten your legs is sometimes a long process. Shortened hamstrings shouldn't keep you from forward bending, though. Bend your knees so that your torso rests on or near your thighs. Then slowly begin to straighten your legs, stretching the hamstrings. Keep your back straight.

Trouble Spots in Jumping Sun

Q: I tried it and collapsed on the floor! I don't think I have enough strength to do it.

A: The best way to build strength for a specific task is to just do the task. In the beginning skip Hover Pose, jumping from Intense Forward Bend into Dog Stretch. Then swing into Upward Dog Stretch and back to Dog Stretch. Jump forward and finish the cycle.

Q: Jumping jars my body.

A: Practice jumping like a cat on a hot tin roof . . . *spring!* Don't pounce.

Q: I collapse in Hover Position.

A: Practice Hover Pose by itself with knees on the floor for a while. Gradually use your knees less and less, hovering more and more. Side benefits? Beautiful "pecs," chest muscles.

Q: If I manage to get from Hover to Upward Dog Stretch, I collapse again in the second Hover. After that, there's no way I can push up into Dog Stretch.

A: Skip the second Hover for awhile. Swing from Upward Dog Stretch into Dog Stretch.

When you're ready to add Hover back in, practice the second one with your knees on the floor. Then push up into Table Pose and back into Dog Stretch. Voilà! You've got it!

Jumping Sun Practice Plan

- Start this series after you have increased your stamina with Sun Swings. Jumping Sun is a demanding system of movement.

- Do one cycle of Jumping Sun after your sets of Sun Swings.

- Gradually increase the number of Jumping Suns according to your ability.

- Make your own modifications. Jump back into Dog Stretch instead of down into Hover Pose, skipping a more difficult part of the Jumping Sun. Then do your swings from Downward Dog to Upward Dog Stretch.

- Implement the Big Three Principles: Tip and Tuck, Cosmic Sandwich, and Dynamic Duo, safeguarding and strengthening your back.

- Synchronize your movements with your breath, just as you do in swimming, running, skiing, and walking.

- Intersperse the Jumping Sun with the Sun Swings. It's like incorporating sprints into distance runs.

KEY IDEA: Use the Jumping Sun to increase your cardiovascular output. It demands training and endurance to maintain a steady pace, gradually increasing the number of cycles.

Here's to you and Sun Power! Once you're hooked on it, you won't leave home without it.

RELAXATION POSE (SAVASANA)

This pose helps you to develop the ability to become fully relaxed, yet conscious. It trains the body in stillness, the mind in alert quietness and teaches systematic release of tension throughout the entire body, permitting full extension and alignment.

- Sit on the floor in Staff Pose.
- Bend your knees, and keep the soles of your feet on the floor.
- Place hands behind your hips, palms down. Tuck your fingers under your buttocks.
- Lean back on your elbows, your chin in, chest expanded, and shoulders away from ears.
- Rest the back of your pelvis on your hands.
- Press your feet to the floor and gently push your body backward, hips sliding over hands, until your whole back, pelvis to shoulders, rests on the floor.
- Your head comes to the floor, chin tucked, back of neck elongated.
- Slide your hands out from under your hips and turn palms up.
- Extend your arms outward about 15° from your sides.
- Press your whole body downward into the floor—your feet, lower back, and the back of your neck and head. Feel your spine elongating.
- Exhale and relax.
- Extend first your right leg out on the floor, and then the left. Your feet, knees, and thighs turn outward (Figure 3.114).
- Watch your thoughts come and go with warm detachment.
- Turn your attention to yourself. Noises and activity around you fade in and out of consciousness. You are aware of them but you have nothing to do with them.
- Imagine that time and space are fading away.
- Your breath flows in and out, in and out. Listen for the stillness at the end of each exhalation.

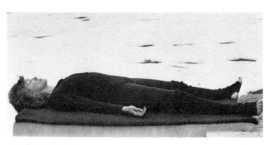

FIGURE 3.114

- Feel the tension leave your body, from the crown of your head to the soles of your feet.
- Your face is soft and tranquil, your eyes heavy and still.
- Relax the tongue in your mouth; your jaw is heavy.
- Arms and legs feel soft and heavy.
- Your hands and feet melt into the floor.
- Become very still and listen to the internal sounds of your body: the rhythmical beat of your heart, the breath flowing in and out, your stomach and intestines, and your brain with its thought waves and deeper consciousness.
- Rest for a while in the space and expansion within you, a center of peace and wholeness. The whole is greater than the sum of its parts.
- Now it is time to slowly awaken again. Stimulate the nerve impulses to every cell in your body.
- Begin to stretch your fingers and toes. Stretch them wide apart.
- Roll onto your side in Fetal Pose, knees to chest, hands cushioning your head.
- Take a few rhythmical breaths.
- When you're ready, come to a sitting position.
- Sit for a few moments with your legs and ankles crossed, spine straight, head centered, and hands on knees. Retain the centeredness you experienced in Relaxation Pose. May the force be with you.

WINNING-EDGE WORKOUT PLAN

Don't be surprised at the feeling of expansiveness and extension you get from your workout. Your muscles have just been to school, learning about their new length and strength. They're all pumped up and feeding back data to your brain and spinal column. Your joints are well oiled, and they know a little more about their range of motion.

The result is a new perspective on what you can do. You are sharply alert, relaxed, and confident. You can deal with life's intricacies and emergencies. Great return on your investment of time! When you think you haven't got the time, review the alternatives. Do you want to rust out or wear out? Consider the time you spend preparing meals and eating every day. Dare yourself to put equal time into your Winning-Edge Workout!

If you don't regularly meet with yourself every day, you lose your center. You become scattered and ineffective.

Undercover Exercise extends your workout throughout the day. Make a personal contract with yourself that you'll commit at least 15 minutes a day to your Winning-Edge Workout: 10 minutes of Trainers and 5 minutes of Relaxation Pose. See the Winning-Edge Workout Plan to help you plan your practice. Gradually increase your time in the Trainers or increase undercover activity for the day. Incorporate your choice of aerobic activity before or after the Trainers, or any time during the day.

Suggested time for each pose or Trainer is an estimated time for getting into and out of the pose and for working in the pose. You can gradually increase or decrease the time in each pose, adapting the workout to your body and to your own needs. You are the authority. Mix and match the poses to give you *at least* a 15-minute Winning-Edge Workout. Don't forget to include 5 minutes of Relaxation Pose at the end of the workout.

Back and Body Trainers

Standing Poses		Sitting Poses		Floor Poses	
Mountain Pose	1 min.	Staff Pose	1 min.	Supine Tip and Tuck	1 min.
Coffee Break Stretch	½ min.	Sit Back	30 sec.	Cat-Cow Pose	1 min.
One-Legger	1 min.	Boat Pose	30 sec.	Cobra Pose	30 sec.
One-Legger Twist	1 min.	Doorknob Squat	1 min.	Desk Pose	1 min.
Flying One-Legger	1 min.	Bellows Squat	30 sec. – 1 min.	Knee-to-Chest Squeeze	2 min.
Tree Pose	2 min.	Seated Forward Bend	1 min.	Supine One-Legger	1 min.
Standing Eagle	2 min.	Supine Jack Knife	1 min.	Head to Knee	1 min.
Back Press	1 min.	Sitting Eagle	1 min.	Huggy Pose	1 min.
Mogul	½ min.	Eagle Balance	30 sec.	Turkey Pose	2 min.
Hot Dog	1 min.	Bound Angle	1 min.	Cat Stretch	1 min.
90°Forward Bend	1½ min.	Sitting Leg Stretch	2–3 min.	Child's Pose	1 min.
Dog Stretch	1 min.	Roofer's Twist	1 min.	Neck Press	1 min.
Triangle	2 min.	Sitting Twist	2–3 min.	Head Roll-Up	1 min.
Split-Leg Forward Bend	2 min.			Torso Curls	1½ min.
Fencer's Pose	1 min.			Easy Back Twist	1½ – 2 min.
Runner's Lunge	1 min.			Supine Eagle	30 sec. – 1 min.
Warrior	1 min.			Supine Torso Twist	2–3 min.
Intense Forward Bend	1 min.			Hover Pose	15 sec.
One-Step Backbend	½ min.			Upward Dog Stretch	15–30 sec.
Standing Half Bow	1 min.			Downward Dog Stretch	15—30 sec.
Ballet Bow	1 min.			Handstand	1 min.
Spread Eagle Forward Bend	1 min.			Half Headstand	1 min.
				Half Shoulderstand	½ – 1 min.
				Relaxation Pose	5–15 min.

Hanging Poses

Bar Hang	1 min.
Hanging Bow	1 min.

Sun Power Series

Sun Swings (one set)	1–2 min.
Jumping Sun	15–30 sec.
For aerobic workout	20–30 min.

Model Workouts

30-Minute Workout
For Problem Backs

Supine Tip and Tuck	1 min.
Knee-to-Chest Squeeze	2 min.
Supine One-Legger	1 min.
Turkey Pose	2 min.
Head Roll-Up	1 min.
Torso Curls	1½ min.
Desk Pose	1 min.
Cat-Cow Pose	1 min.
Runner's Lunge	1 min.
Dog Stretch	1 min.
Door Knob Squat	1 min.
Back Press	1 min.
Standing Eagle	2 min.
Bar Hang	1 min.
Supine Torso Twist	2–3 min.
Relaxation Pose	10 min.

60-Minute Workout
For Strength and Stamina

Sun Swings	10 min.
Jumping Sun	5 min.
Triangle	2 min.
Split-Leg Forward Bend	2 min.
Fencer's Pose	1 min.
Warrior	1 min.
Standing Bow	1 min.
Ballet Bow	1 min.
Handstand	1–5 min.
Half Headstand	1–5 min.
Half Shoulderstand	1–5 min.
Bar Hang	1–5 min.
Sitting Leg Stretch	3 min.
Sitting Twist	3 min.
Supine Torso Twist	3 min.
Supine Eagle	1 min.
Sitting Eagle	1 min.
Eagle Balance	1 min.
Seated Forward Bend	1 min.
Relaxation Pose	15 min.

15-Minute Workout

Cat-Cow Pose	1 min.
Cat Stretch	1 min.
Child's Pose	1 min.
Huggy Pose	1 min.
Sit Back	1 min.
Bound Angle	1 min.
Easy Back Twist	1 min.
Knee-to-Chest Squeeze	2 min.
Head Roll Up	1 min.
Relaxation Pose	5 min.

Alternate 15-Minute Workout

Sun Swings (one set)	1–2 min.
Tree Pose	2 min.
Triangle	2 min.
Fencer's Pose	1 min.
Warrior	1 min.
Sitting Leg Stretch	2 min.
Relaxation Pose	5 min.

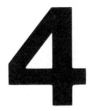

4

What Goes On Behind Bathroom Doors?

What we have to be is what we are.
Thomas Merton, "Extemporaneous Remarks"

This is your Clark Kent act. Take your Winning-Edge Workout into the bathroom. Ten minutes later you come out from behind closed doors a new person.

Your *approach* is the key. It's the mind-switch we dealt with in Chapter 2. Is it going to be the same old mindless routine, or will you throw the switch? You can do more than you think in the next ten minutes. You will pay respect to the person you are and the best that you can be. It's like putting your house in tip-top shape.

Stand in front of your bathroom mirror. Face the mirror squarely, or roundly if you're overweight! Stand in Mountain Pose. Remember the jingle that can take you through your entire day: *Plant your feet, balance your pelvis, lift your sternum, relax your shoulders, center your head and keep growing up.*

Look yourself right in the eye. Get acquainted with who you are this morning. Say "Hi" to yourself, and then you're ready to wash your face.

WASHING YOUR FACE

Place your hands on the washbasin. Using the Fulcrum-Lever Concept, walk your feet and hips backward until your spine is parallel to the floor. Give your face 50 splashes in Suspension Bridge or 90° Forward Bend, your first hamstring stretch of the day.

Support yourself with one arm on the washbasin. Step forward with your right leg and do Split-Leg Forward Bend as in Figure 4.1. Feel the additional stretch to your front leg. Now change legs. Bring the right leg back and the left forward. Repeat the pose.

If these stretches are hard for you first thing in the morning, do Standing Eagle. If that's too hard for you, go back to bed!

Standing Eagle
Bend your knees and drop your hips. Bring your right leg around the left knee and hook the foot around the left calf. Press it against the outside of the left calf or just place your

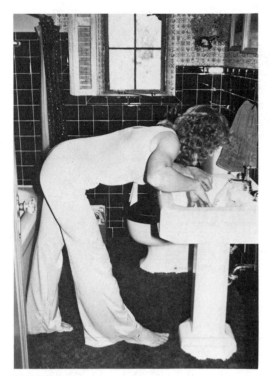

FIGURE 4.1

the washbasin throughout this exercise until you're sure of your balance. Look around for a chair, stool, pile of books, magazines, or any kind of ledge in the bathroom. Lift your leg and stretch it out in front of you, resting your foot on the prop. If you're very limber, you can place your leg on the wall, counter, or washbasin (Figure 4.2). The aim is to have both legs straight, but you can vary the pose by bending your lifted leg, as in Figure 3.1.

Bring your torso erect again and do One-Legger Twist (Figure 4.3). It's the first waistline nipper of the day. With both legs straight, turn your torso *toward* the lifted leg. You can hold onto this leg as you turn. Balance your pelvis. Lift your sternum. Turn and look over your back shoulder. Keep your earlobes parallel to the floor. This is a great neck stretcher.

Turn and face the mirror again. Level your shoulders and look yourself right in the eye. Now turn your torso to the left. Use your

right foot on the floor beside the outer left foot. You'll feel a stretch in the hips and sacrum. That should feel very good to you. It relieves strain to the lower back. You'll find this exercise a helpful posture throughout the day, especially when you can't find a bathroom!

Change legs, wrapping the left leg around the right. This gentle squeeze increases the venous return of blood from the legs to the heart.

Congratulations, you're through washing your face. Stand in Mountain Pose. Look at yourself and see how fresh and alive your skin looks. Now you're ready to brush your teeth.

BRUSHING YOUR TEETH

With toothbrush in hand, do One-Legger. It's a good hamstring stretch. Keep holding onto

FIGURE 4.2

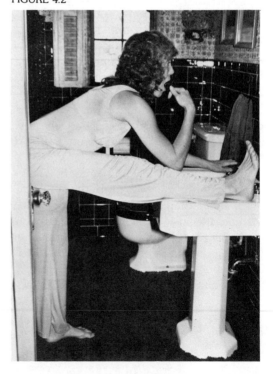

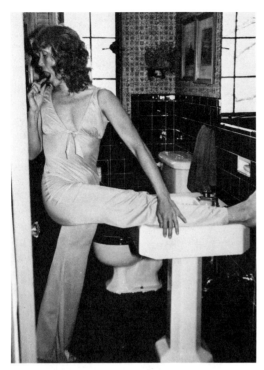

FIGURE 4.3

Each bathroom offers different workout possibilities. I finish my workout swinging from Dog Stretch to Upward Dog Stretch. The lavatory and tub in Figure 4.4 are just the right distance apart and can hold my weight!

THE SQUAT THAT COUNTS

Here we go . . . the squat that counts! The squat brings a rich blood supply to the entire pelvic region. This area is responsible for removal of wastes and toxins. Since it also houses the sexual organs, it often becomes congested with tension, worry, fear, and feelings about our sexuality. Muscles, organs, and every cell in the body must have a rich blood supply to function at their best. Tension and fear contribute to poor muscle function and groggy organs!

Consider the time and energy we spend eating compared to the time and energy we spend eliminating what we eat. We have a habit of hoarding things, including food! We

right hand to push *away* from the lifted leg, as you turn in the opposite direction. With your free hand, hold on to the wall, doorjamb, towel rack, shower stall, washbasin, toilet top, or whatever you can. Look over your left shoulder. It's fun to do a forward bend here to get an early morning groin stretch. You'll become an ambidexterous toothbrusher by the time you're through. Come back to center. Lift the opposite leg and twist again toward, and then away from, the lifted leg. Enjoy the sensational surge of energy you get from these twists.

You can do a One-Step Backbend and Tree Pose while you finish brushing or flossing. Stand tall without tension. Feel yourself held up like a marionette, a line of energy from the top of your head drawing you upward. Stretch the front and the back of your body equally in Cosmic Sandwich. Feel long and svelte early in the morning; keep that feeling with you throughout the day!

FIGURE 4.4

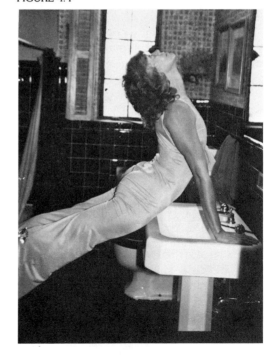

perish in our rubbish if we don't take care of our disposal system! There's only so much food you can pack in there before the plumbing system backs up! Then you reach for a laxative. You're not alone, judging by the variety of laxatives on the market. What are your alternatives?

I often think of the little lady who came to me in desperation because she simply couldn't go to the bathroom without her daily laxative. After two weeks of practicing her Winning-Edge Workout, with special attention to the squat, she could finally give up those laxatives. That's one of the benefits of the squat.

Stand in Mountain Pose. Grasp the door knobs, one in each hand, for the Doorknob Squat (Figure 4.5). Make sure that the doorknobs and the door can hold you.

Bend your knees and drop your pelvis as much as you can. If you can't go all the way down into the full squat, just stay at whatever level is workable for you. Work your legs and feet. Keep your buttocks off the floor. No sitting down on the job! Great exercise for skiers and dancers.

Stay in the squat and practice abdominal breathing. This brings movement, energy, and life into the pelvic area. Be sure to exhale completely and don't overdo it.

Here's the fun part! As you exhale, push down on your feet and lift into a standing position. Inhale. On your next exhalation, lower your hips into the squat position again. Let yourself hang with your hips about one inch off the floor. Up and down you go like a teeter-totter on a playground. Keep your breathing rhythmical and full, coordinated with your body movements. This will exercise your lungs and massage your internal organs.

Now close the door and see if you can squat without holding onto anything. Just in case, hold on to a prop. Use the edge of the toilet, vanity, or bathtub until you've had some practice. Exhale, bend your knees and

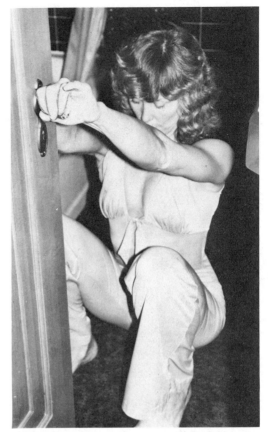

FIGURE 4.5

drop your hips as far as you can. Stay about one inch from the floor.

See if you can let go of your prop and maintain your balance. If you fall backward, hold on to your prop again, but don't hold on to your breath! Keep breathing. If you can go all the way into a full squat keeping your balance, you can do the Bellows Squat from Back Trainers, Figure 3.58. Feel the bellows drawing the air in as you inhale, and squeezing the air out as you exhale. As you do this rhythmically several times, practice Pelvic Floor Pull-Ups.

Since you're in the bathroom anyway, check the strength of your pelvic floor muscles by stopping and starting the flow of your urine. When you do this successfully, you are doing very subtle and important muscle work that can affect the health of your urogenital organs. Review Pelvic Floor Pull-Ups in Back Trainers, if necessary.

Don't be inhibited about exercising this part of your body. Throughout the book, you'll be encouraged to use Pelvic Floor Pull-Ups wherever and whenever you can. It's a secret source of strength and power. Who knows, maybe that's what Mona Lisa was smiling about so mysteriously!

You're all warmed up now. You are ready for whatever you need to do: shower, dress, go to the office, or go on to your Winning-Edge Workout. Nice way to warm up for your workout.

SHOWER DELUXE

Hit the showers! Enjoy the sensuality of the water playing on your skin. What a great feeling. Turn around several times and let all your muscles get nice and warm. Then start your shower workout by turning your back to the shower head for One-Step Backbend (Figure 4.6A). Place your right foot behind you and stretch your arms up toward the ceiling. Reach backward for the shower head or push against the wall above and behind you.

Turn on Core Power and Dynamic Duo. The warm water will help you to fully contract your core muscles and experience a wonderful sense of length and suppleness in your body. Look upward, but beware of falling water! Switch legs and do the backbend with your right leg forward. If your back hurts in the backbend position, review backbending under Dynamic Duo in Chapter 3.

Now rotate your pelvis-spine forward in the Split-Leg Forward Bend, reaching for the wall in front of you (Figure 4.6B). Relax your buttocks as you rotate forward, keeping the lever straight. Put your hands on the wall or anything you can hold on to. You can always press your hands against the wall. Feel the warm water massaging your back. Keep your hips level and legs working. Can you feel the stretch of your hamstrings and calf muscles? Switch legs and do the pose with the opposite leg forward.

Go into Suspension Bridge by bringing the forward leg back, feet parallel to each other. As the water warms your muscles, stretch the sides of your body equally. Stretch your legs and entire length of your spine. Hang out there for a while. The warm water will encourage your body to give up its tightness and rigidity.

Hold on to something in the shower for One-Legger. Stand on a rubber mat for safe footing. Carefully lift one leg and rest it on a ledge, or press that foot against a wall. You can keep both legs straight or bend the lifted leg. You'll feel the stretch to both legs. Now bend forward from your hip joints, over the lifted leg. Remember to apply the Fulcrum-Lever Concept. Make this a Two-Way Stretch. Then lower the leg and repeat the stretch, standing on the opposite leg. You've done this One-Legger at the washbasin and you'll find yourself doing it again and again, everywhere you go.

From the One-Legger, go right into One-Legger Twist. Turn your torso 90° to the side of the lifted leg. Place your hands on the wall at shoulder or chest level and push against the wall, increasing the twist. Twist from the navel and pelvis. *Use all the walls and resistances in your life to enhance you capabilities!*

You may have trouble keeping your balance with one leg up. Try the twist with both feet on the mat, one leg forward, or one leg back, as you did in Split-Leg Forward Bend. Twist 90° to the side of the forward leg.

Holding on for safety, do Tree Pose (Figure 4.6C). Soapsuds may make your legs

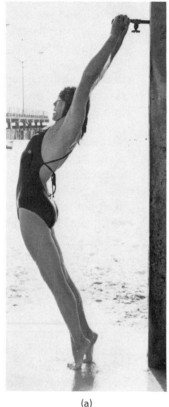
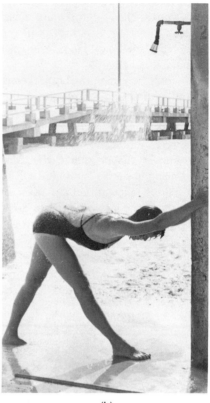

FIGURE 4.6

(a)   (b)

slippery, so please be careful. This is a great pose to do while you wait for conditioners to do all those wonderful things they're supposed to do for your hair.

Go from Tree Pose to Mogul (Figure 4.6D) for a great leg workout. Stay down as long as you can. It does wonders for your back, legs, and abdominals!

You will use the shower bar, door, or side of the stall for the next twist. Check and make sure that whatever you're using can hold some of your body weight. I remember the morning I ended up with a not-so-secure shower bar in my hands. Now, hold on to the bar and drop your hips a little bit. Bend your knees and stretch down and away from the bar. Don't hang your weight on the bar, but use it to increase your stretch.

Now hold on to the bar for the Bar Hang Twist. Stand with one leg up on the wall or tub, as in One-Legger Twist. Twist toward the lifted leg and then away from it. This gives you a great stretch in the arms and shoulders. Lift the opposite leg and repeat the twist. Keep your hips level. The warmth of the water will boost your turning power.

The Neck Stretch is good for pains in the neck! Turn around so that the water is on your back. This is an easy stretch to do while you shampoo your hair. Clasp your hands around the back of your head and draw your head down toward your chest. Keep your pelvis balanced, sternum lifted, and body upright. The only thing you're pulling down is your head. Let the water massage the back of your neck and feel the nice long stretch. As you draw your head upward, resist the lift of your head by pulling downward with your

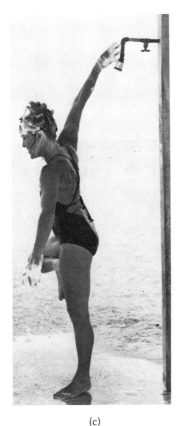

(c)

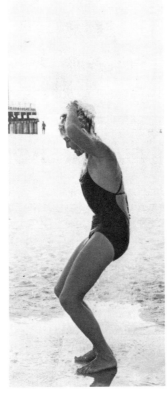

(d)

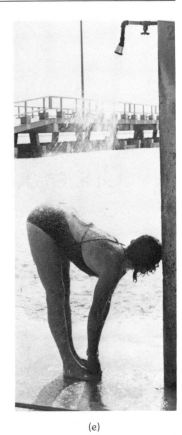

(e)

hands. When the head comes back to center, release your hold and relax.

You're about to imitate a gargoyle, one of those animal-shaped drain spouts on roof gutters. This exercise is similar to Intense Forward Bend. Moving from the fulcrum, rotate the pelvis-spine out and downward, hands reaching for toes. Bend your knees if you need to. Grasp your big toes with your index fingers and just hold. Feel the water running down your back, helping the stretch. Try not to drown. If you can straighten your legs, you're in luck. Your back will become a water slide, and your chin becomes the spout (see Figure 4.6E).

Tips for a Shower Deluxe

1. *Sing.* Pretend that you are in the Kennedy Center and sing to the last row in the balcony.

2. *Brush.* Use a loofa sponge or natural bristle brush to shine your hide.

3. *Invigorate.* Finish with a cold shower. You're tough! Look out, world!

4. *Massage.* Your skin loves to be rubbed with oil or lotion. Give it a polishing.

You'll never know just how great a shower workout can make you feel until you try it. Add your own ideas to these and come up with a luxurious home spa treatment!

5

Undercover Antics on the Go

Life is either a daring adventure or nothing.
Helen Keller, *The Story of My Life*

Travel is a perfect cover for Undercover Exercise. With "ears on" and spyglass in hand, Undercover Agents are on the go. They are traveling the highroads and backroads of intrigue and adventure. The lure of faraway places has more appeal to most of us than going to the store, but for an Undercover Agent, there is just as much intrigue in going to the store as there is in traveling to foreign climes. So whether you're home or away you can audaciously or covertly do UEs wherever you go.

It takes courage and imagination to recognize the potential in every situation. Remember that you can't do in a strange city what you haven't practiced in your own backyard.

THE JOURNEY

Whoever you are and wherever you go, you have to cover ground to get there. The only unknown is how. The unknown has always been the allure but also the stress of traveling.

Even if you choose to evade the rigors of traveling, you still need to go somewhere, sometime. You can benefit from this chapter as much as the adventurer who relishes the intrigue and uncertainty of being on the go.

Let's see what kinds of UEs can ease everyday traveling. Then we'll investigate the possibilities of UEs on long-distance ventures.

Commuting

Walking   Most of us have to travel to work. Public transportation has become a major problem in many cities. It is a mystery that we can travel to the moon, but here on earth we still can't get people to and from work.

Most of us are fortunate enough to have two working legs. Those who don't are quick to remind those of us who do how fortunate we really are! The undercover adventure of the man in Figure 5.1 is obvious.

As you walk, use the principle of Cosmic Sandwich. Make it an aerobic exercise. Rather than resent your walking environment, find beauty in it. Observe the people passing

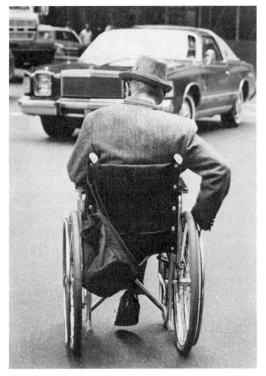

FIGURE 5.1

sides or carry equal loads on both sides of your body.

Walking and carrying added weight can be a great advantage if the weight is balanced. It increases your workout and can burn extra calories. Carry your own luggage and baggage whenever possible, but don't let it weigh you down. The gentleman in Figure 5.2 is on his way home with his briefcase and shopping bag. He has the advantage of carrying weight on both sides of his body, but he is missing out on a UE. If he used Cosmic Sandwich, with balanced pelvis and squared shoulders, he could carry himself in alignment and get a good workout!

If it's impossible for you to walk to work, you can get your walking in by walking briskly

FIGURE 5.2

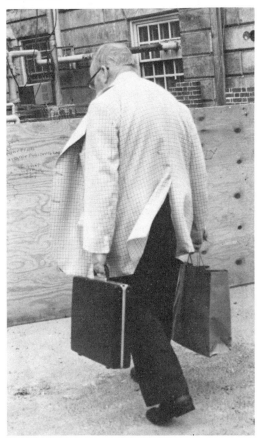

by. Watch their body language. Be alert to everything that's happening. Learn to sense the intent of those around you. You can't always be correct, but you can avert many potential dangers by being observant. Watch, listen, and sense. Stay clear and centered. This will train you in sizing up situations quickly and in making decisions based on the facts. Put fear in its proper place; it's an alarm system. Respond to the alarm with keen observation.

Walk briskly and *don't look weak!* Carry yourself with purpose, strength, and direction. You may have to carry a big stick, hat pin, whistle, or whatever else gives you a margin of safety. Stay alert and let fear alert you rather than blind you.

As you walk, notice which shoulder usually shoulders the load. If you carry your briefcase, purse, or bag on the same shoulder all the time, you become lopsided. Change

to your bus, car pool, or subway. This can be part of your aerobic workout.

Erase overanxious and time-pressured thoughts like "I'm going to be late" or "I've got to make this train." They are the seeds of heart attacks. You don't need them. Play a song, jingle, or verse in your mind as you hustle for it. Use hurrying to your advantage by turning it into a good workout.

Bicycling   Maybe you're one of the lucky ones, like my husband, who can bike to work. You have the advantage of getting your regular aerobic workout going to and from work.

My Uncle Siegfried has never owned or driven a car. In Germany that isn't so unusual. Every morning of his working career, he biked across the city at 4:00 A.M. and then back home again in the afternoon. He biked to work in rain, snow, or shine.

Uncle Siegfried is incredibly strong. He survived the concentration camps of Russia and walked home from Siberia. Nothing daunts him except air travel. He gets where he needs to go keeping his feet or wheels on the ground!

Running   Some people are literally running to work! It's another great way to do your aerobic workout enroute to work. It requires planning. You'll need a shower at work, or a sponge bath and a change of clothes. Your colleagues will be happier about working with you!

Be alert to pollution patterns. Don't hesitate to wear a mask if you are in heavily polluted areas. Learn the wind patterns and the time of day when the air is cleanest.

If you walk, run, or bike to work, go early, before the heavy rush of traffic and automobile fumes. Avoid streets with stop and go traffic. Find the safest routes. They're usually more scenic anyway. A little winding around circumventing heavy traffic will make your run more interesting and give you alternate routes.

There's a great new style afoot in our big cities. People are wearing running shoes with grey flannel suits. The latest status symbol is an athletic bag in one hand and an attache case in the other! It says you're working out before or after hours or during your lunch break. Fitness and vitality vibrate right through the fibers of your suit. Madison Avenue can't sell that—you earn it!

Subway   Some of you have to go underground to get around. It's a whole different world underground! I was terrified in London, intimidated in Stockholm, sardined in Philadelphia, awed in Washington, D.C., petrified in New York, and lost in Boston. Three little words went with me all the way: "Don't look weak!"

It's always reassuring to see other people doing UEs, such as the man doing a UE squat while he waits for the train in Boston (Figure 5.3).

As a keen Undercover Agent, you've got your "ears on." You are watching, listening, and sensing everything around you. You can tell right away whether overt or covert UEs are in order. Intruding on someone else's

FIGURE 5.3

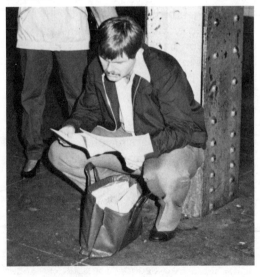

space or showing off your skills in public? Tacky! Be discreet! Do whatever UEs you can without a ruckus. You can always do breathing exercises or Pelvic Floor Pull-Ups.

You can get by with a one-arm Bar Hang (Figure 5.4) almost anytime. Alternate arms and get that great stretch in your arms and shoulders. Another version of the Bar Hang has the same shape as the Boat, Staff, or Dog Stretch. Hang from both arms, drop your seat, and keep your legs and back straight. With a One-Step Backbend (Figure 5.5), you can work tension out of your shoulders and practice Dynamic Duo at the same time. If you can do Undercover Exercise on this New York subway, you can do it anywhere!

Continue your workout as you leave the underground. Do a One-Legger on the exit gate (Figure 5.6). Glide into the Runner's Lunge. Try to switch legs and do it on both sides if you get the chance. That'll depend on whether you've got a crowd behind you or not. Even if you get in just one leg stretch, "Something's better than nothing," says my good friend Hans Shacklette.

Bus Watch people waiting at the bus stop. Some sit, some shift from one leg to another, some even run in place. If you're not satisfied with sitting but feel conspicuous running, then do Hot Dog (Figure 5.7), a powerful but inconspicuous UE, and one you can get by with

FIGURE 5.4

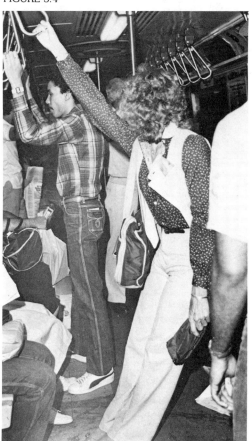

FIGURE 5.5

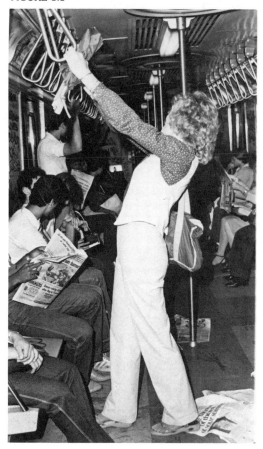

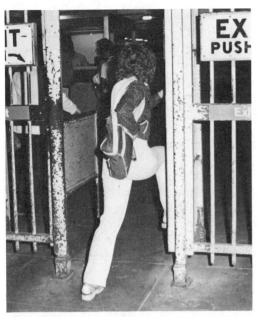

FIGURE 5.6

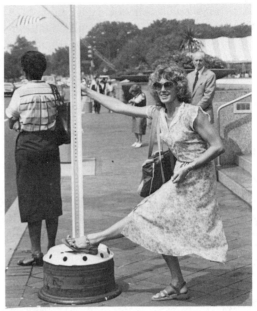

FIGURE 5.7

in so many places. Dynamite for your legs! By the weekend you'll be ready to hit the slopes. If you want strong, conditioned legs, do Hot Dog everywhere you go.

Play with variations of the Standing Eagle. It's easy to do and lends itself to many standing situations. All you have to do is flex your knees, put one knee in front of the other, and dip your pelvis and knees (Figure 5.8). It's a great back saver! I don't know what I'd do without it! You can lengthen your spine and tuck your pelvis without much ado.

The Standing Bow is a good addition to your standing UE repertoire. Stand on one leg and bend the opposite knee to 90°. This gives you a good stretch in the hip flexors and quadriceps muscles in the front of your thighs. You can grasp the ankle for even more stretch. Be aware of your alignment. Don't jut out your hip. Keep your spine and torso in Cosmic Sandwich. Swaybacks will have to remember to tuck the pelvis to do this pose safely. The One-Legger is another indispensible UE. Do it on ledges, stairs, or any prop. It's a good waiting-for-anything exercise!

It takes raw courage to get on a crowded bus . . . unless you like becoming a sardine. You never know who's pinching you! If you get stuck standing, at least you can do a Bar Hang (look again at Figure 5.4) from the handrail or practice Mountain Pose. Breathing exercises may be very difficult to do with people's perfumes, cigarette smoke, and body odor all around you, but here's an exercise you can practice anytime. I call it Empathy Observation. It requires no exchange of words. It's a warm detachment that just observes. It is done by imagining yourself on the inside, looking out through another person's eyes. You have the advantage of seeing another's point of view. This is an art that demands a lot of practice. You can become very skilled at being "one with" or pacing another person. You find a deeper self that is universal in all of us. It is an essential art for all Undercover Agents. There is no better place to practice Empathy Observation than on a crowded bus, plane, or train.

If you have a seat on the bus, here are some UEs that can get you to work fresh and

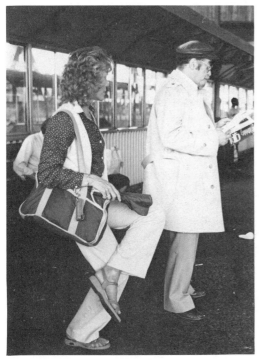

FIGURE 5.8

alert or revive you on the way home. Do the Back Press against the seat. It's amazing what it can do for your back. Breathe into your back and feel it stretch and lengthen against the seat. Avoid the usual slump! It only makes your back worse and puts pressure on your lumbar discs. It also does nothing for a tired, dejected spirit.

Knee-to-Chest Squeeze or Knee Lifts will get you breathing rhythmically again and elongate your back, releasing tension in your tight back muscles. (See Figure 6.2 in Chapter 6.)

A Sitting Twist (Figure 5.9) brings a fresh blood supply to your weary back and shoulders. Tension is replaced with energy! Cross your knees or keep them together. Hold on with your opposite hand to the leg or knee of the side to which you're twisting. You can hook your other arm over the back of the seat or press it against the seat. Feel the inches melting off your waistline!

Car Have to drive to work? Car pool if you can. Can you see the possibilities for synchronized twists in the back seat? Knee-to-Chest Squeezes and Double Knee Lifts (Figure 5.10) will work off your morning bagel and cream cheese! If you don't have a fun car-pool group, trade them in! If you can't, you can do your Pelvic Floor Pull-Ups and Back Press all the way to and from work. No one will be wise to what your're doing.

The president of a large company said that by the time he arrived at his office each morning, he'd made himself sick with mounting pressures and tension. I taught him how to do the Undercover Take-off and a variation of Cat-Cow while driving to work. They changed his attitude and his day.

Here's the Cat-Cow he uses. You learned it in Table Pose. Turn it on end, your bottom end. Hold the steering wheel in both hands, or reach for the dashboard or back seat. Expand your chest and tip your pelvis forward as you inhale. Tuck your pelvis and draw your lower ribs inward as you exhale. The rhythmical breathing and movement will

FIGURE 5.9

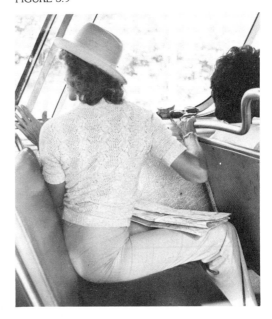

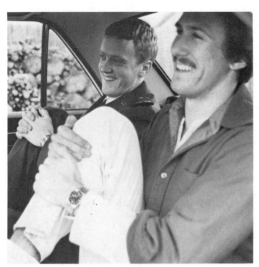

FIGURE 5.10

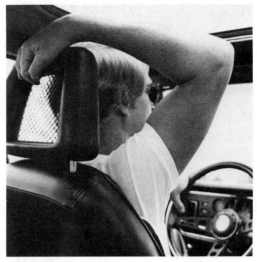

FIGURE 5.11

help you establish a quiet but alert mind that will help get you through your day . . . in style!

Do these rhythmical Cat-Cow movements *without* deep breathing when you're caught in a traffic jam. Idling cars cause a buildup of noxious fumes and you don't want to deeply inhale them. This rhythmical exercise will help you with frustration by giving you something positive to do while you wait! If you are stopped by road crews or traffic jams and get stuck waiting . . . and waiting . . . and waiting, turn off your engine and do your UEs. If it's safe to get out of the car, do a few One-Leggers on the bumper or fender.

Do a variation of Executive Stretch while you're driving. With one hand, reach up and back for the head rest. Use it to help you stretch. Pull your elbow back behind you and expand your chest (Figure 5.11). It gets rid of shoulder and neck tension and makes you more alert. Truckers and other long-distance drivers can really use this UE throughout a trip. Switch hands and repeat the stretch. At stoplights you can use both arms in Executive Stretch.

Long-distance car travel means anything from several hours in a car to days on

the road. Each summer for the last three years, my family has taken a cross-country road trip. Our car was like a little space capsule where we could all be together. No phones or outside activities, nothing to pull us away from each other. We actually were able to be just a family of four for a while! It's a great way to get reaquainted. Sometimes it took a major conference to decide what the majority wanted to do. But after four days there and four days back, we got the hang of conspiring with each other. We ended each trip with a treasury of family memories. Some of them kept us laughing throughout the year.

It was a riot watching the UEs that each family member devised along the way. Chris, our older son, who is 6'4" and still growing, put his long legs through the opening of the sunroof (Figure 5.12). I awoke from a nap to see this huge kid with his feet stuck out the top of the car and naturally asked him what he was doing. "Cooling my heels, Mom," was the answer I got.

You can use the headliner of the car or sunroof to do a reaching stretch, twist in your seat, do Double Knee Lifts, and Executive Stretch. Periodically, take tension out of your neck by pushing one hand against the side of

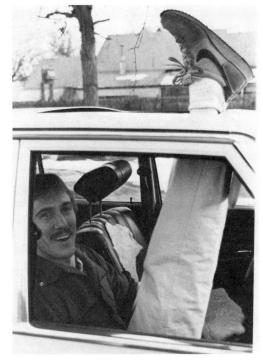

FIGURE 5.12

your head. Resist the push with your head. This strengthens the neck and releases tension.

Pelvic Floor Pull-Ups are as valuable on long-distance trips as anywhere else. They can be a lifesaver for truckers, bus drivers, and other long-distance drivers by keeping the pelvic floor tissues healthy and helping to guard against hemorrhoids, an occupational hazard of people who sit for hours at a time.

My favorite UEs at gas stations are the Hot Dog and the good old One-Legger. Use them as you "fill 'er up."

Motel or hotel pools provide a nice break from travel fatigue. See the pool workout described later in this chapter. It'll revive and energize you again. Every corner of your motel/hotel room is an incredible playground. Your Winning-Edge Workout every morning will keep up your training. Remember that Sun Power is a good aerobic workout in a small space. Use your bathroom

workout (Chapter 4) as often as possible. It'll prepare you for the long days on the road.

Train

I love trains. I'm saddened by the decline of the grandeur and elegance of train travel. But it is still a fascinating and exciting way to go. There's a hustle and bustle in train stations that airports can never match. Grand Central Station in New York City is my favorite. Travelers are dwarfed by that grand domed edifice. They look like ants racing single-mindedly to their destinations.

I even like trying to make a train at rush hour. The feeling of packing into the feeder troughs always makes me feel like mooing. There's a great sense of camaraderie at being jostled around and using your bags as battering rams. Have you ever had someone else standing on the back of your sandals as you try to move? The press of human bodies just seems a natural part of it all. A great place for UEs? You bet! Here's a perfect situation for Back Press (Figure 5.13).

FIGURE 5.13

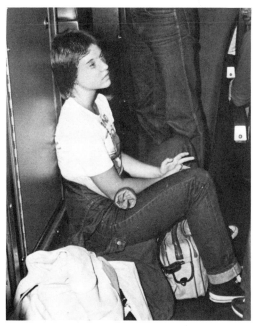

If you are lucky enough to nab a seat, you can workout doing UEs for hours! Pay special attention to your feet, your poor feet! Use the footrest to press against as you flex and point your toes. This helps reduce swelling in your ankles and feet.

The footrest elevates your knees so that they are a little higher than your hips, helping to take strain off your lower back by balancing or tucking your pelvis. Using the footrest also keeps the edge of the seat from pressing into the backs of your thighs and cutting off circulation to your lower legs and feet. Press your back firmly into the seat. Use Core Power to elongate your spine as you exhale. Practice Cosmic Sandwich just as you did in Staff Pose.

Push your seat back and do Boat Pose. You can rest your feet on the back of the seat in front of you (Figure 5.14). The gentleman in front doesn't know that my feet are on the back of his chair. Remember, invading the private space of another person cancels out the benefits of your UEs.

Stretch your legs whenever you can. Your knees are bent most of the time when you travel. Unbend them.

Handling your own luggage on long-

FIGURE 5.14

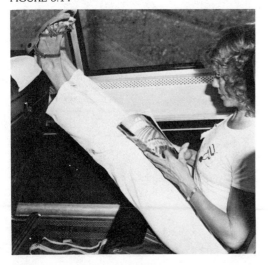

distance train rides is a chance to do some strength training along the way. Don't attempt this if you have a problem back or are not in good physical condition. Call a porter.

One of the benefits of your Winning-Edge Workout is that you become strong enough to handle your own weight, as well as your luggage. Place yourself in a centered position, pelvis tucked and legs slightly bent. Exhaling, hoist your bag onto your bent knee. Juggle it until you have control of the bag (Figure 5.15A). Turn on Core Power! Exhaling, draw the weight close to your body. Inhale, get set. Exhale, go! Lift it up and onto the ledge (Figure 5.15B). Phhhhh, what a load!

You can use that same ledge that holds your bag to help you stretch. Take every chance you get to do a tall, reaching stretch. Hold onto the ledge and stretch upward. Tuck your tail and breathe into it. Practice Dynamic Duo.

The stress and strain of traveling put your back into a very vulnerable state. All it takes is a quick, unthinking, off-centered movement to put a vulnerable back out of commission. Each time you remember to do a UE, you are lessening the stress and strain to your body. You look and feel better as you safely support your spine.

We so often cheat ourselves of the power and energy that really is ours. All the little moments of missed UEs add up to a deficit of energy and zest, a surplus of fatigue and vexation. We miss a lot of lifts that come our way!

Airplane

Walking and bicycling give you a ground-level view of the world. Flying gives you an astronaut's view. Either way, Undercover Agents see the relationships among all kinds of living things. As you observe, you become tuned in to the cause and effect of the universe.

I've learned from my biogeochemist husband that looking at a tiny community of

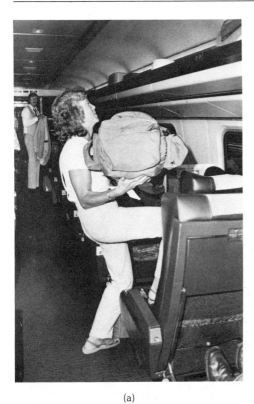

(a)

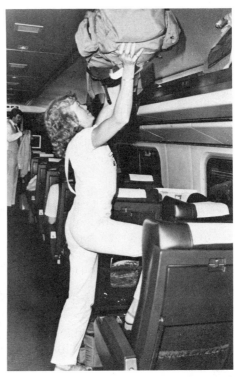

(b)

FIGURE 5.15

plants—a microcosm—is like looking into the universe, the macrocosm. He can see the universe without taking a step.

When you fly, you begin to realize the revolution in understanding that has come from seeing the first photographs of earth from outer space. Your flying time gives you a better understanding of yourself in the larger scheme of things.

When we fly, our bodies don't have the time to acclimate to new time zones and climates as did our ancestors', who traveled slower, by ships and covered wagons. Zip, zip and we're there! Our bodies have to cope with our jet age.

A lot of attention has been paid to the problem of jetlag and how to overcome it. Our circadian rhythms get confused when we are suddenly eight hours ahead or four hours behind. The body can't be fooled. It knows it's not time for breakfast at midnight!

Our bodies have to adjust slowly to new time zones when we travel. But just as the body begins to adjust . . . zip, zip and we're back home again. How can you counteract the effects of speed—the rapid change in time zones, water, food, and culture? UEs!

The three essentials—circulation, alignment, and extention—can do wonders for your ability to adjust to and enjoy your new environment. UEs provide a great way to work out and entertain yourself while on board. You'll arrive fresh and alert! Some airlines have published booklets on how to exercise while aboard. They are excellent helps.

Here are some of the UEs I do while flying. The first thing you'll need to consider is visibility. Will someone discover your undercover antics? You are the best judge of what you can do comfortably without feeling conspicuous. Your skills as an Undercover Agent are needed here.

Two of the most inconspicuous UEs are Staff Pose and Back Press. Stretch and extend your legs as much as you can. Press your back firmly to the chair. Try this with the seat in both the upright and reclining position. Breathe quietly and rhythmically as you do your Pelvic Floor Pull-Ups. You can do this while you read, eat, or visit with the attendants. No one will be the wiser except you. You'll be sharp, alert, and full of fun!

How about some fresh air? Great chance for a UE! Reach up and fiddle with the air valves (Figure 5.16). Take a long time and breath into the stretch.

Getting a little braver? Do the Executive Stretch. Expand your ribcage. Lift your sternum and elongate your spine. Do the Two-Way Stretch from sternum to tailbone. Breathe rhythmically and feel the expansiveness of your chest. (Figure 6.1, p. 122.)

Animals usually stretch when they change position, so why should you be shy? Just remember that everyone would like to do what you're doing . . . or at least reap the benefits. So be brave! From Executive Stretch, keep your fingers laced together and stretch arms and palms up toward the ceiling. Take your time. You appear self-conscious only if you are. Be deliberate and smooth in your movements and breath. Feels great, right?

Your back can get mighty tired and sore when you travel—from a combination of hauling bags, rushing, standing, and sitting for incredible lengths of time, and just plain anxiety.

Do your back a favor and take a few moments to do Knee-to-Chest Squeeze. A few rhythmical breaths in this position do wonders for your back and your peace of mind. I often draw both knees to my chest, place my feet on the edge of the seat, and

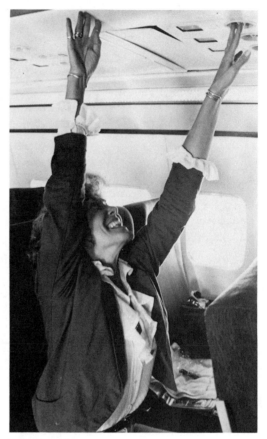

FIGURE 5.16

"buckle up for safety." The seatbelt around my ankles lengthens my back and relieves some of the stress of sitting.

If any of the UEs are too overt for you, then modify them. You can always prop your feet up on your carry-on lugguage or whatever you can find. This raises the legs, lengthens your back, reduces stress and helps with swollen ankles and feet.

If you eat too much, drink too much, and sit inactive for the entire flight, you will arrive feeling and looking lousy! UEs can help you work off that excess indulgence and the trimmings around your waistline.

Do Knee Lifts in Staff Pose. Start with one at a time, then try Double Knee Lifts. Keep your back pressed firmly to the seat.

Hold both knees up toward your chest as long as you can, breathing rhythmically. Press down with your hands on the edges of your seat to help you lift your legs. Do these as often as you can. They work out excess tension and can keep you looking terrific in your new bathing suit!

The Sitting Twists are waistline trimmers. They increase circulation to your spinal column. Cross your legs or keep them parallel to each other. It's the same kind of twist that you can do on the bus or in the car. Point your knees straight ahead and turn your torso 90° to the side (Figure 5.17). Your hips will turn slightly with your torso. Take your time in the twist and hold it as you breathe. I always pretend to be looking down the aisle and then out the window. I don't think I could survive without these twists!

When you sit for long periods of time without exercising, your legs stiffen and cramp, your feet swell, and you get "butt fatigue." Stretch out your legs as often as you can. Walk up and down the aisle, or go to the lavatory. Be aware of the flight attendants and don't get in their way! Stay put if they're serving in the aisle. You can work out in your seat a little longer.

There's usually a line of people waiting to use the lavatory. Do Standing Eagle while you wait in line. Someone may ask you if you need to be next!

Stand at the window and watch the clouds. Combine Hot Dog with a One-Legger, a terrific way to de-tensify your legs (Figure 5.18). I wouldn't exchange the Hot Dog for any amount of money! I think it's a great tension workout and leg shaper. Follow Hot Dog with Standing Bow, a thigh stretcher, or do a Split-Leg Forward Bend. You can do just a simple One-Legger if that's all you get by with undetected. This is a test of your skill! Remember that your skill as an Undercover Agent is in maneuvering yourself into positions that stretch you. Every situation demands a review of tactics!

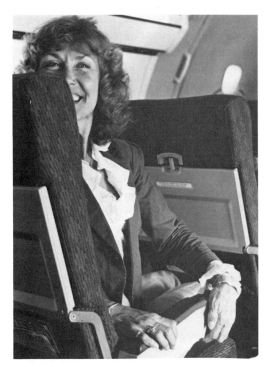

FIGURE 5.17

FIGURE 5.18

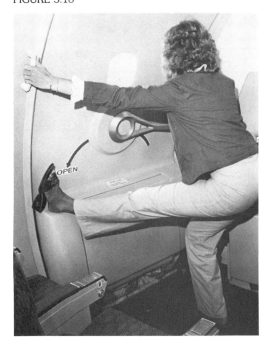

Watch children! They naturally do UEs all the time. The boy in Figure 5.19 innately knows how to make his back feel good. He's elongating his lower back in a Back Press against the wall.

At least in the lavatory you've got privacy . . . for a few moments anyway. Take time to do the Diamond Gait, an absolutely indispensible part of your repertoire. You can increase your pulse rate and get your system going with the rhythmical arm and leg movements. Do the same opposite arm and leg movements as you do in a brisk march. Bend your arms and knees and march in place (Figure 5.20). You've only got a small space, so lift those legs and swing those arms! Sing a song like "Stars and Stripes Forever" to get it going. Right arm and left knee up . . . then left arm and right knee up. If there's no one wait-ing to use the lavatory, do the Diamond Gait for 3 to 5 minutes; cut it short if someone's waiting.

I hate to mention the unmentionable, but it's very important. Your mother warned you about toilet seats! Listen to her for a change. Every public toilet is a chance to practice the Mogul or Half Squat. No fair touching! Great for your legs.

The possibilities for UEs are limited only by your imagination, strategy, and *training*. You *cannot* be creative and inventive without regular training in your daily Winning-Edge Workout. Don't neglect it!

What do you do for travel tremors? A lot of vacations and trips are spoiled by fear and frustration. The "What ifs" cause a lot of anxiety. Delays and disrupted plans cause a lot of anger and disappointments. Murphy's law

FIGURE 5.19

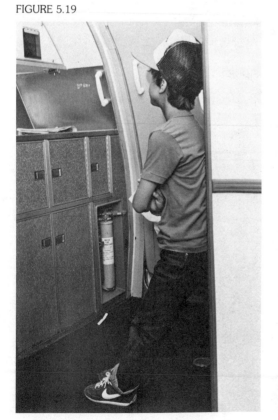

FIGURE 5.20

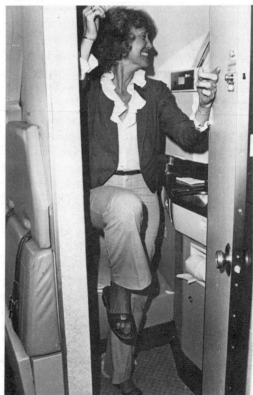

comes into play again: "Everything that can possibly go wrong, will go wrong." Cartoon it!

Breathe rhythmically and play a video in your mind. Go over all the mental "What ifs": What if I miss my connection? What if I get sick? What if there's a hijacking? What if the place crashes? Consider your fears about the most final "What if." Think of all the alternatives you have with each "What if," and then put them to rest. If the worst happens, you're prepared; if it doesn't you're spared!

Enjoy! Your trip is a high adventure, a romantic intrigue that features Agent 00? Wow! That's you! Sing a song in your head that keeps your spirits light and free. But above all, *use your secret resource!* Do UEs wherever you go. Not only will they keep you strong, alert, and alive . . . but the rhythmical breathing helps release natural tranquilizers in the brain (they're called endorphins). They'll help you feel calm and give you a natural high. The best feeling of all is the feeling of well-being. Keep those endorphins flowing!

Delays

These lines from C.S. Lewis sum up the Undercover Agent's philosophy of delays and interruptions: "The great thing, if one can, is to stop regarding all the unpleasant things as interruptions of one 'own,' or 'real,' life. The truth is of course that what one calls interruptions are precisely one's real life [8]."

Rather than curse the turn of events, use them! How many of you have regreted piques and pouts that spoiled a vacation or a trip? It takes absolutely no skill to pout or complain. It takes incentive and inventiveness to see what you can do with delays and interruptions. The opportunity to do UEs is one interruption you can welcome, for UEs interrupt tension and put you at ease again!

Airline terminals offer you the chance to make sensible use of "down time." There are plenty of spaces and places for working out. Go to the restroom and do a 20-minute Diamond Gait. I've done Sun Swings in boots

and full dress in the restroom. All you have to do is wash your hands afterward. Nothing else needs to touch the ground. Handstands are great UEs when you need a Bottoms Up and don't want to get anything but your hands dirty. You'll be surprised at how much better you feel after getting a little more oxygen to your brain.

When you're out in the waiting room, be more discreet. Find a place where you won't be bothering anyone and do a Back Press (Figure 5.21). It'll get you breathing rhythmically again as it calms you and gets rid of the kinks!

Train terminals offer you a different set of circumstances. Their restrooms often are not the best places to spend your layover time. Bathrooms are likely places for wanderers who need sobering, a nap, or a little extra cash. Check out the rest of the terminal. You can always rent a locker for your baggage and go for a brisk walk. If you feel the area around the station is not safe for walking, then do UEs

FIGURE 5.21

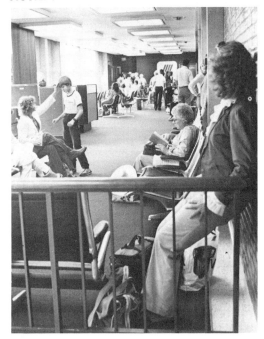

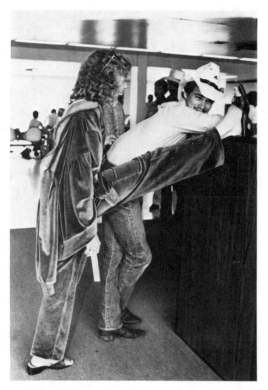

FIGURE 5.22

standing in the station or sitting on a bench. There's always something you can do (Figure 5.22).

Car breakdowns and their accompanying delays can be scary, frustrating, and even funny. They are the stuff memories are made of. Thinking ahead and preparing for contingencies help reduce the chances of those emergencies. But even the best laid plans can go awry. Little towns, country farmhouses, roadside cafes, and garages often become the places of refuge.

You all have your own stories to tell. Some include surviving under the worst possible circumstances—hurricane, flood, or blizzard. These are the times that test your mettel. China bowls shatter when hit. Clay holds the impression of every poke and punch. Yeast dough rolls with the punches and becomes more vigorous with the kneading. The

more the dough raises, the more air, light, and life it holds. Roll with the punches!

Accidents do happen. If you are observant and drive defensively, most of them can be averted. But sometimes, no matter how carefully you drive, you can get hit right out of nowhere!

I was crossing a busy intersection near my home when a drunk driver, traveling 55 mph, crashed through the red light into the passenger side of my car. I was almost across the intersection, and two lanes of stopped cars hid her approach. I don't remember the impact. They tell me that my car was catapulted into the air three times, flipped over in midair, and came down on the roof, spinning around 180° degrees. Kope, a paramedic, was the first person on the scene. She had seen the accident through her rearview mirror. She found me dangling upside down from my seatbelt, my head and arms swinging like a pendulum. I remember the feeling of being upside down. It was just like being in a Bar Hang or a Bottoms Up UE. My body was not afraid. I remember thinking, "Isn't this interesting." Then Kope's voice snapped me out of my euphoria. I unfastened my seatbelt and slithered through a broken window, using Cobra Pose to get out of the car. (See Figure 5.23A−B.)

All my training paid off. It had survival value. I am grateful to be alive and to have been spared the misery of severe injury. The structure of our old '69 Saab, the seatbelt, the surprise impact, and the strength and flexibility of my body helped save my life. The accident gave me a firm resolve to do whatever I had been spared to do.

The story of the Kent family is very similar. All five of them have come to our classes. Sue was driving home with her two daughters when they were hit by a car and slammed into a telephone pole. There *were* injuries, but the three of them made rapid recoveries. Sue feels that she speeded her recovery by being in excellent condition at the time of the acci-

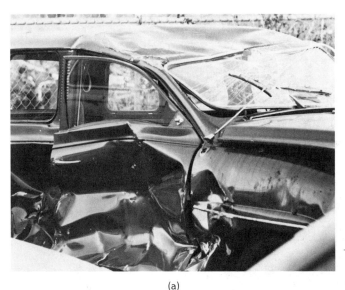

(a)

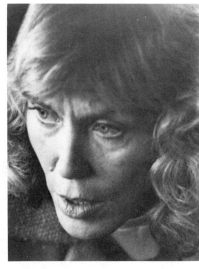

(b)

FIGURE 5.23

dent, and by doing whatever UEs she could do during her down time. She can't do everything yet, but she's back in full swing, Sue style! She's helping her own healing by consistent, persistent practice.

The training pays off in times like these! You can fall back on your resources. Sue said her best resource was being able to walk all by herself in a stiff-legged Dog Stretch to the bathroom. No bedpans for Sue! It's those little things in life that count!

VACATIONS

Here you are on location. It's your vacation! You've been saving your time and money all year and here it is . . . your big splurge!

Many of us gravitate to water for fun and relaxation, so here is a whole section on UEs in the water or beside it. Then we'll investigate UEs that save your back and legs while you sightsee and tour.

Water Work and Play

There is nothing like water to increase your circulation, aid your alignment, and help with extension. One student said after the whirlpool work on our latest retreat, "I've never felt better! Isn't there some way to do this every day?" Yes! Do your shower workout (Chapter 4), bathtub workout (Chapter 8), or do these UEs in a hottub or whirlpool at home.

This group of students (Figure 5.24) is working on standing poses. Warrior Pose practiced in warm water encourages lengthening of the back and work in the legs. You can get even length on both sides of your torso as you reach upward. Feel your pelvis-spine lever as a unit supported by the water. Squeeze your thighs together and close the groin. Use the advantage of the warm water to get more rotation in your back leg. Think of leveling your hip joints and turning the hip of the back leg as far forward as you can. Incorporate Dynamic Duo to extend your spine.

All the standing poses are fun to do in a whirlpool. For partner work, adapt the workout in Chapter 8 to water. Be careful not to overdo your workout in hot water. You can accomplish a lot in a very short time with

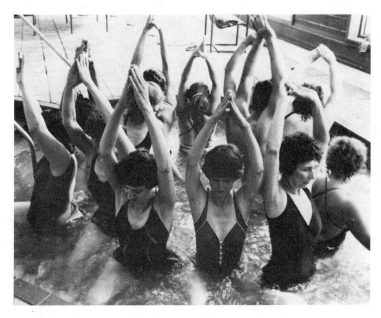

FIGURE 5.24

warm water as your ally. Be sure to replace lost fluids and electrolytes. You've been perspiring and can easily become dehydrated.

Sit quietly for a while with your back pressed against the wall of the pool. Cross your legs in Tailor Pose. Do Double Knee Lifts or Knee-to-Chest Squeeze. Then practice Boat Pose, working your abdominals and thighs. The water supports your legs and makes it easier for you to lift both legs. Turn on Core Power!

Train for backbends with a chest expander in the water. Do a One-Step Backbend or Coffee Break Stretch, grasping the railing behind you. Be sure to tuck your pelvis. You'll be able to stretch your hip flexors like you've never stretched them before!

Holding onto the railing, do a Flying One-Legger (Figure 5.25). Your body is supported by water and it's surprising how different the exercise feels when you have the water helping you with your alignment.

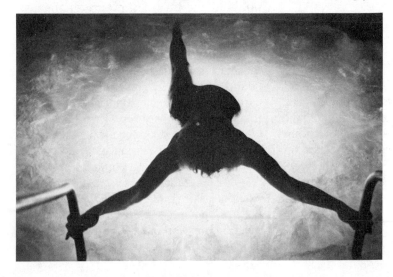

FIGURE 5.25

No hottub or whirlpool? Work in cooler water, as shown in Figure 5.26A–D. Augment your health and beauty treatment with a One-Legger. Use the stairs that lead into the pool. Place your foot on the first, second, or third step, or prop your foot on the railing (Figure 5.26A).

It doesn't matter what medium you find yourself in. The same training principles apply whether you're on land, air, or water. You've practiced them diligently in your Winning-Edge Workout so that your exercises can be a natural part of every new environment or activity.

Play on the railings the way you did as a kid. You can hang on with both hands, wrap your feet around the bar, and swing like a hammock. Then do Ballet Bow and Standing Bow.

Sit on the stairs or ledge and do a Sitting Twist (Figure 5.26B). Use the water and rail to help you turn from the navel. Keep your legs firm and allow your hips to turn slightly with the twist.

On deck, do Desk Pose (Figure 5.26C).

There are some simple UEs you can do with your flippers before flipping through the water. Intense Forward Bend and Sitting Forward Bend are fun to do with your extremely big feet! Then hold onto your flippers and get a good leg stretch (Figure 5.26D).

Do a Relaxation Pose out under the sky. This is one of your best Undercover Exercises. It looks like you've died from the outside, but you're really coming alive on the inside!

So much for pools and hottubs. Let's go to the sea! A vacation by the sea is a dream come true for many people. It offers sun, sand, salt, tan bodies, and the roar of waves. But most important, it offers a chance to communicate with yourself, each other, and the natural world. It's a time of renewal—in Anne Morrow Lindbergh's words, "a gift from the sea." The creatures we encounter remind

FIGURE 5.26

(a)

(b)

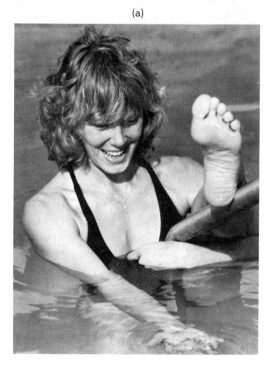
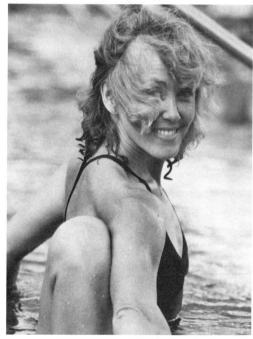

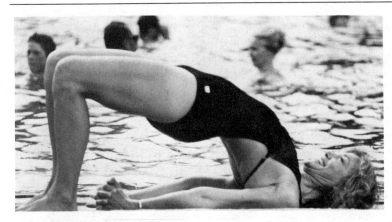

FIGURE 5.26 (cont.)

(c)

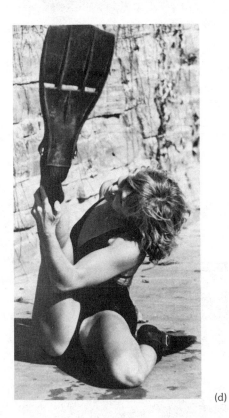

(d)

breath . . . coming in and going out. Feel your breath swell and crest, the stillness of the hang-time, and then the breaking of the waves upon the shore as they recede to the source. So moves your breath. Be still and know. . . .

Watch a child playing in the sand. Observe the naturalness and spontaneity, the complete absorption. There are many ways of meditating, reflecting, and contemplating. Sometimes it's hard for adults to be as unself-conscious as a child, but in complete contemplation, the ego-self dissolves and we are a part of something bigger than ourselves.

In the early morning hours before the rest of the crew awakens, take some time for a workout on the beach. The sand gives you new footholds.

Stretch upward and greet the sun in Sun Power (Figure 5.27A). The sun is a symbol of the light and energy of your center. Then go into Intense Forward Bend (Figure 5.27B). Feel your roots in the earth.

Slide one leg back into Runner's Lunge (Figure 5.27C). Reflect on your connection with the earth and the firmament above you.

Exhaling, slide the forward leg back into Dog Stretch (Figure 5.27D). Inhale into Upward Dog Stretch (5.27E), and then back into Dog Stretch (5.27F), Runner's Lunge (5.27G), Intense Forward Bend (5.27H), and up to greet the sun (5.27I).

us of our connection with other forms of life, our interrelatedness with all living things.

Plan some quiet time for yourself. Find a place to sit quietly and absorb your surroundings. It requires no special mantras or rituals. Open your mind and your being to new insights. Let the waves remind you of your

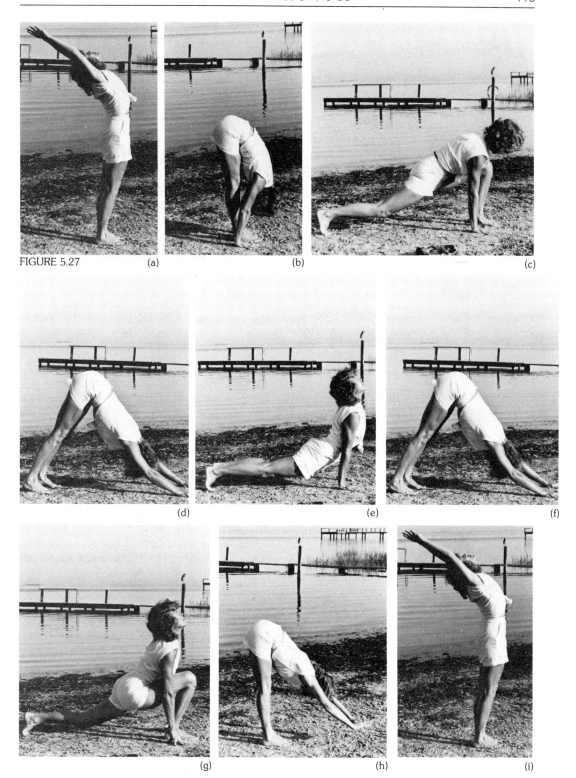

FIGURE 5.27

(a)   (b)   (c)

(d)   (e)   (f)

(g)   (h)   (i)

Combing the beach and riding the waves is a tremendous workout for body and soul. "Wade in the water, children" is the injunction given us in the old spiritual. Wading and walking is an enormous workout for your feet, legs, and abdominals. Leap and play like a child. Notice your impressions in the sand. Use this time to check out your foot placement.

Join in the fun of a water sport. It'll test your strength and courage! Have you ever tried wind sailing? Even a well-trained athlete can stand on a board with firm, strong legs and in seconds end up with legs like jelly.

Here I am fighting the sail (Figure 5.28). This is a good example of how your training prepares you for whatever you want to do. Hauling up the sail is something you can count on doing often, especially as a novice. What a workout for every ounce of your body!

Now look at a pro do it (Figure 5.29)!

FIGURE 5.28

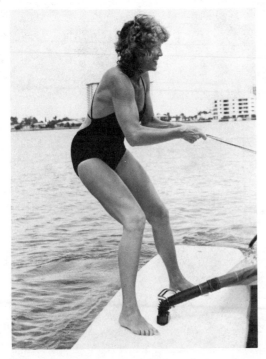

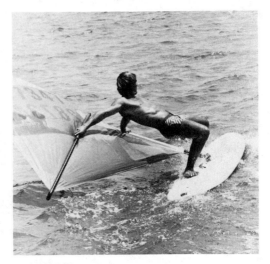

FIGURE 5.29

This is Mark Robinson, president of West Coast Water Sports, Inc., in Clearwater Beach, Florida. Windsurfing is Mark's work and play. He gave us a breath-taking show of grace, elegance, strength, and stamina. UEs provide a good foundation for a sport like this. This is the pay-off for consistent, persistent training.

Backpacking

Backpacking and hiking are increasingly popular ways to see the countryside. They provide an intimate experience with the natural world. Get properly fitted shoes and pack, and then load them both for good weight balance. Practice Mountain Pose with your weighted pack on your back. See if you can spread your toes in your boots.

Use the hipstrap around your hips to help you tuck or balance your pelvis as you walk. It's a terrific aid for keeping spinal extension. I learned this on a field trip with my husband. I wore a fanny pack as a weight to keep my lower back in extension. It helped me to end my day in a beautiful way: *no backache!* I did all the UEs I could possibly do along the way, and the weighted pack was an asset. Imagine the Two-Way Stretch you can do with *extra* weight stabilizing your hips.

Carrying a heavy pack, or even just your own body weight, up a steep mountain slope can be very discouraging. My husband taught me the Rest Step, which got me through many a climb. It spared me the gasping fits of stops and starts!

Practice the Rest Step on a hillside. You need the hill to carry you along. Take small steps. Bring your right leg forward and put all your weight on it. Rest your left leg as you swing it limply forward. Then put it down a short step forward of your right. Shift your weight to the left leg and repeat the procedure.

You can climb this way forever, taking small steps at a time. Synchronize your breathing with your steps. It becomes a meditation. Before you know it, the crest of the hill is at your feet.

Sightseeing and Touring

Vacations often involve a lot of tiring sightseeing, and that can make everyone cranky and irritable. But sightseeing gives us new insights into who we are and what we share in common with each other. As we go back to our roots, we experience the courage and determination of our ancestors.

Figure 5.30 shows the ship where the Boston Tea Party took place. As I stood on deck, I tried to imagine the thoughts and feelings of the people who took part in this historical event.

National monuments and historical markers remind us of the great people and events of our past, of the drama of human sacrifice and dedication to a cause. They challenge us to new visions of ourselves and our part in history.

Figure 5.31 shows our great lady of the harbor! Did you know that she is doing a One-Step Backbend? Notice her planted feet, balanced pelvis, and centered head. She's growing up!

Seeing the Statue of Liberty for the first time, I imagined how my father must have felt as a young man catching sight of her standing

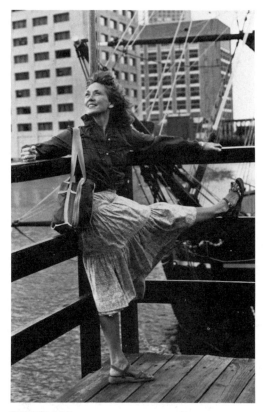

FIGURE 5.30

in the harbor. Like countless others, he came seeking his fortune. He found it, but not quite in the way he had planned. As a clergyman and hospital chaplain, my father has enriched the lives of many, as well as his own.

Personal pilgrimages take us to our roots. They bring past and present together. They give us time for reflection and send us home with new perspectives.

Whether you tour by surrey or bus, apply all the tips you've learned traveling in the car, airplane and train. Surreys, especially with fringe on top, are an excellent way to go back in time. The clop-clop-clop of the horses' hoofs on the pavement and the swaying of the carriage give you a sense of timelessness. A Double Knee Lift or Sitting Leg Stretch enroute can revive flagging spirits (Figure 5.32).

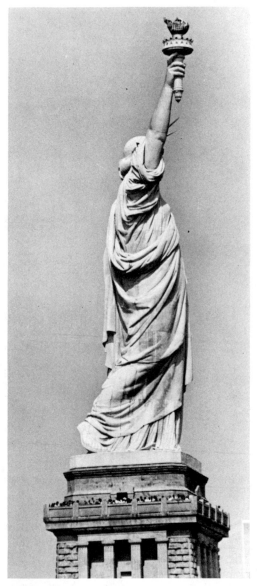

FIGURE 5.31

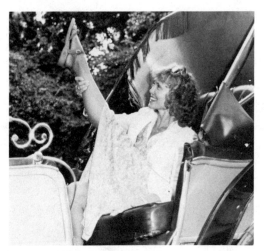

FIGURE 5.32

FIGURE 5.33

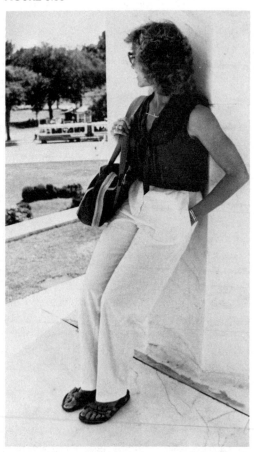

Use walls to rest against and do the Back Press (Figure 5.33). Practice Cosmic Sandwich as you breathe rhythmically in the pose. You'll take that tension right out of your back!

Use bars and railings for Bar Hangs and twists. The young man in Figure 5.34 just naturally and spontaneously does Bar Hangs

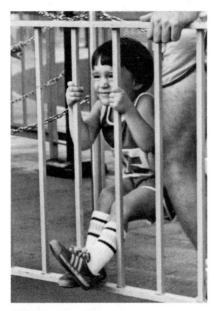

FIGURE 5.34

while he waits for his ride at Disneyworld. You can, too (Figure 5.35A–B)!

Roadside rest stops not only provide a place to rest but some of them provide beauti-ful views and historical markers about the countryside. Suspension Bridge is a wonder-ful stretch after sitting for a long time (Figure 5.36). Roadside markers make excellent props.

Be alert and aware and stay alive! Prac-ticing UEs all along the way helps you per-ceive and respond quickly to the realities of your environment. They keep you monitoring the information that pours into your senses every minute. They keep you poised, clear, and centered.

A workout in the beautiful natural set-tings of our National Parks can be a warm memory in the months after you return home. A Triangle on the canyon rim at Mesa Verde National Park was especially fun for me (Fig-ure 5.37). It brought back memories of nights on the mesa listening to coyotes howling up and down the canyon. My husband did his research work here, and we spent a lot of time climbing around the canyon walls with our sons on our backs.

It was important for me to spend some-time by myself away from the crowds. I

FIGURE 5.35

(a)

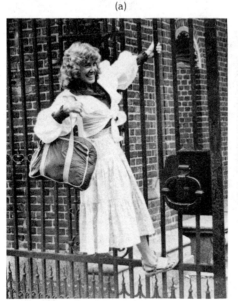

(b)

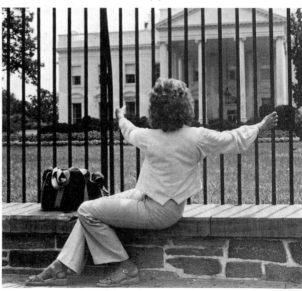

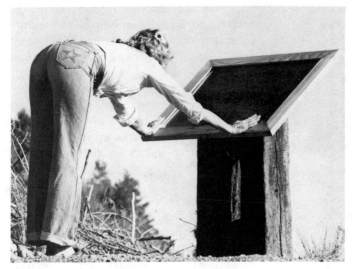

FIGURE 5.36

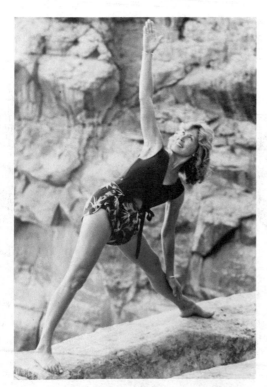

FIGURE 5.37

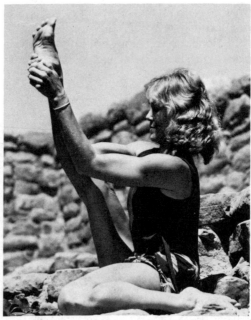

FIGURE 5.38

worked out alone, looking down the canyon (Figure 5.38). There I was able to better understand where I had been, how far I had come, and where I was going.

There is a special feeling here, a connection with the "ancient ones," the Anasasi. Twenty-two years ago, I sat at a mano-matate similar to the one in Figure 5.39, pretending to be an ancient one grinding corn. Suddenly I felt my heels fit into the sandstone wall be-

hind me, into the worn places rubbed away by the heels of another more ancient mother.

Now my sons have grown and in the intervening years, I have become a little more ancient myself! Vacations are times for getting away, for putting things in perspective and then coming home refreshed and ready to get on with whatever you've chosen as your mission.

FIGURE 5.39

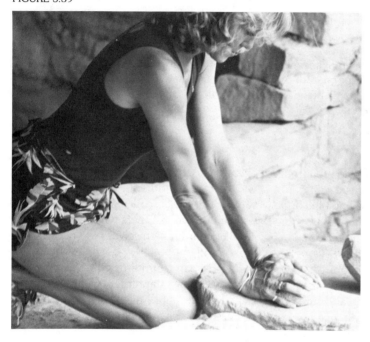

6

Undercover Agents on the Job

An excellent plumber is infinitely more admirable
than an incompetent philosopher. The society which
scorns excellence in plumbing . . . and tolerates
shoddiness in philosophy . . . will have neither good
plumbing nor good philosophy . . . Neither its pipes
nor its theories will hold water.
John Gardner, *Excellence: Can We Be Equal and
Excellent Too?*

He was only 5′5″ tall, and a little stooped from pushing a broom for so long. His disguise included a railroad engineer's cap and blue and white stripped coveralls. He bound up our wounds, listened, cajoled, laughed, and cried with us. He left an indelible mark on everyone who went in and out of that school. His title was custodian. It was a good cover. His mission was counselor, peacemaker, and support crew! It was my first teaching job away from home. This man showed me the reality of what I'd learned from Mom and Dad: It doesn't matter so much *what* you do, but *how* you do it.

Undercover Exercise celebrates the excellence and integrity of everyday work. Every task is worthwhile. The spirit, talent, and experience of each person make the wheels go round. As an Undercover Agent, you influence everyone you contact. If you settle for anything less than your best, we all lose!

In this chapter you'll see other agents using the cover of everyday tasks as powerful

exercises. Ask yourself what you can do that will inject your job with excitement and the sense of an undercover mission. You'll find yourself drawn to others who are looking for excellence from themselves . . . and recognizing it in others.

UEs can counteract the occupational hazards of sititis, standitis, burnout, and inefficiency on the job. Let's investigate how you can use these powerful tools for changing tact or keeping your course. Incorporate these UEs into your sitting, bending, lifting, or reaching on the job. Learn about the pause that refreshes.

THE OCCUPATIONAL HAZARDS

Sititis

What is sititis? It's a pain in the butt! All of you who sit for hours at a time get this dis-ease. Secretaries, computer programers, switchboard operators, long-distance drivers, writers, lawyers, clerks, lab technicians, scientists, anyone who has to sit for long periods of time knows about sititis. It's the hardest thing to stand! The symptoms are neck, shoulder, and/or back pain, restricted breathing, swollen feet and ankles, hemorrhoids, and mental and physical fatigue. Worst of all, it's a continual struggle to keep your backside from spreading out . . . and out . . . and out!

Here's a prescription for treating sititis. *Sit in a chair that fits you,* one that supports your lumbar curve. Remember what you learned about the design of your spine? Your chair should help you maintain the normal curves of your spine, as you do in Cosmic Sandwich.

Cushions can help. If you don't have a chair that's right for you, create one. Put a flat, firm cushion behind your hips and lumbar curve. You should be able to feel your back pressing against it for support.

Your feet should rest completely on the floor, just as they do in Mountain Pose. Make sure there is space between your thighs and edge of the seat. Ideally, your knees should be slightly higher than your hips to lessen strain on the lumbar spine. Place a stool or pile of old telephone books under your feet, especially if you have short legs.

KEY IDEA: Sit as often as possible in Staff Pose. You'll breathe better, feel better, and look better.

Work at a desk that fits you. See if you can place your arms on the desktop and place your hands on the typewriter without lifting your shoulders. Beware! Dis-ease starts here. If you're continually lifting one arm higher than the other or hunching your shoulders, you are asking for headaches, eye strain, neck pain, back strain, and crankiness.

You'll probably be able to adjust your chair more easily than the level of your desk. Put your Class A detective skills to work here. Figure out the cause and effect of the movements you make over and over again throughout the day. Do you continually twist to one side? Is one arm/hand held higher than the other for any length of time? Check your environment. What kind of conditions do you work in all day—lighting, air conditioning, drafts, associates? Check your body position and see how often you stay in that same position.

You may discover the cause of that daily headache or pain in the neck. One of our students who types all day said she finally tried sitting with her legs crossed in Tailor Pose on the desk chair. Her back and neck pain gradually went away and she went home less tired and less irritable.

Kope had been editing this manuscript on the word processor day after day for weeks. She developed severe headaches behind her right eye. She can't see the *E* on the eye chart without her contacts, so anything threatening her eyes terrifies her. When she almost fainted from the pain one night, we took a few minutes to go over cause and effect of the problem. Step by step we traced Kope's normal work day, body positions, symptoms, and anything we could think of that would cast light on the sudden continuous headache. Aha! Everyday, all day, she was turning from the console to the right to read the manuscript. She propped her right elbow on the desk to make notes and then twisted her head to the left to read the machine. Result? Strain to the eyes, neck, shoulders, back, and morale. The lighting was inadequate and she kept the window open, creating a draft around her neck. After soaking in a hot bath, massage, simple UEs, and a complete overhaul of her working conditions and body positions, *no headache!* It left as quickly as it came . . . but not without leaving an impression!

When you have solved the case of proper chair, desk, and working position, adopt this motto, *squirm.* Move around a lot. Wiggle, squiggle, jiggle, and giggle!

The easiest and most natural UE to break the cycle of stress build-up in your neck, shoulders, chest, and back is the Execu-

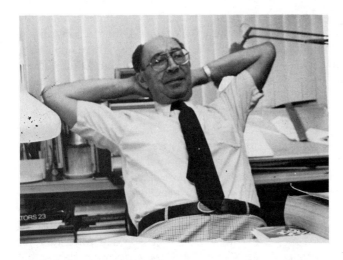

FIGURE 6.1

tive Stretch. This UE got it's name during my regular TV presentation of Undercover Exercise on Denver's KOA "Noonday" show. I was working with the host, Morris Jones, in the chest expander when I noticed how expansive and confident he looked. I told him he looked like a top executive. That's it! The Executive Stretch.

Figure 6.1 shows one of Prentice-Hall's art directors, Hal Siegel, using the stretch to work out the kinks and take some good full breaths. Taking a moment to lean back over the edge of your chair expands not only your ribcage but your productive time as well.

Anyone who spends long hours at a desk knows how hard it is to get and stay fit. Figure 6.2A—C shows Norman B. Pester, CPA, doing the Knee-to-Chest Squeeze, a hamstring stretch, and a twist during his desk work.

Leg and/or Knee Lifts do wonders for stomach tension. If there isn't enough room to lift your legs, then lift your knees like you do in the Bar Hangs. It's a great way to firm those abdominals beneath the cover of your desk.

Remember the Coffee Break Stretch in Chapter 3? Do it sitting at your desk. Reach back behind your chair and clasp hands or a tie. Take your tie off first. You'll live longer! When you want a bit of a break, turn

around and straddle the back of your chair. This Chair Straddle gives you a good groin stretch. If you can, rest your chest against the chair and let your arms and head hang over the back of it. This provides an absolutely incredible release for your back. Find an armless chair that you can use for this UE. You'll love it!

Now sit in your chair like a regular person! Do Staff Pose. Hold on to your elbows and go into Seated Forward Bend. Stop at a 90° position to lengthen your back. Then go into the full Seated Forward Bend. Use this UE to treat brain and butt fatigue.

Now stand behind your chair or desk and do Flying One-Legger. It helps to halt that spreading backside and gives you strong, firm buttocks. Then try the Triangle to banish inertia. If you can't get going on a work project, Triangle will get you started.

My favorite Bottoms Up UE in the office is the See-Saw. Stand facing the back of the chair. Pad the back of the chair if you need to with a towel, sweater, or coat. Rest the area just above your pubic bone on the edge of the chair back. Bend over and hold on to the outer edges of the seat or the armrests. Don't tip the chair! Press your elbows into the back of the chair. Exhaling, lift one leg at a time until you're balanced over the chair. If you

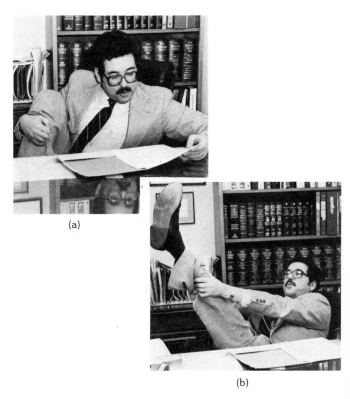

(a)

(b)

FIGURE 6.2

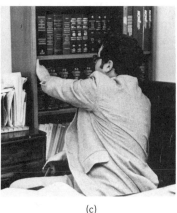

(c)

can, lift both legs together, bringing your head and chest over the seat of the chair. How's this for getting a fresh blood supply to your brain? If you can't lift your legs, just hang over the chairback in a modified Dog Stretch. Feel the effects of this upside-down UE on your mind and body. When you're ready, stand and continue business as usual. Your energy and mid-afternoon exuberance will be remarkable!

Do a few One-Leggers standing beside your chair while you're on the phone. The One-Legger Twist is just a breath away . . . and so is a better outlook and brighter spirit!

Sit in your chair again and take a Relax-

ation Break. Refer to the Pause that Refreshes section later in this chapter.

You've just found out that you can turn your office into a health club! What a workout! Just five minutes of UEs on your chair and under your desk refreshes, awakens, and rejuvenates your entire being. Back to those reports with a renewed sense of energy and vitality.

It's harder to turn the cockpit of an airplace or the driver's seat of a bus or a semi into a health club, but people do it everyday! It's the best-known cure for sititis when you have to keep on sitting.

In Figure 6.3, one of the United Airline

pilots is sneaking a UE with the Executive Stretch. The other is doing a Neck Stretch. How they do their job affects the safety of thousands, so staying alert, clear, and competent is naturally a high priority. Increasing the blood supply to the brain and spinal column by twisting and squirming brings extra oxygen and nutrition to those vital areas. Any flight warrants UEs, but especially long transoceanic flights.

Some of you have to sit through a lot of meetings. They are usually too frequent, too long, and poorly organized. You have to sit there like a nice boy or girl when everything in you wants to take flight. UEs are the magic that can make such meetings bearable. *Squirm!* If you sit still for too long, your brain goes to sleep . . . as well as your feet, your arms, and almost everything else. If you really want to hear the speaker, squirm to keep your brain awake. Any good teacher or speaker knows that a listener's attention span is often less than one minute and no more than three;

then his or her mind is off on its own capers.

Double or Single Knee Lifts can increase circulation and relieve stiffness. Keep your eyes focused on the speaker and sneak in a few casual twists now and then. Don't forget your secret Pelvic Floor Pull-Ups. They can help you stay centered, observant, and clear of mental discussions with yourself. They also are fun to do when you're extremely bored!

Everyone has something to say, something to teach you. Merlin the magician turned that into magic. So can you. Use Empathy Observation (Chapter 5). Put yourself in the leader's place. Understand, or stand under, what others are thinking and feeling. This strategy is effective in friendly and unfriendly encounters. It's also in your own best interest to know what your competitor is thinking. Extrapolate. Apply what you've learned to new problems. Your experiences will help you process new information.

Your Winning-Edge Workout gives you

FIGURE 6.3

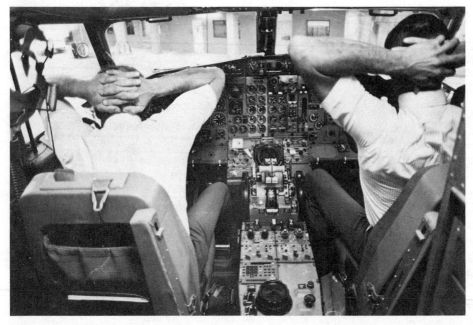

daily training in noticing, observing, and being aware on all levels at once. You'll be amazed at how fascinating meetings and encounters can be when you approach them with the awareness of expression, color, gesture, sound, and undercover nuance. You'll find your shyness or terror fading away as you become involved in the dynamics of the people and events around you. What a relief that is! Ah, the burden of self-consciousness!

Telephone meetings can gobble up inordinate amounts of time. Do one UE after another while you're stuck on the phone. Breathe quietly so you don't sound like an obscene phone call.

Confrontations are difficult for some and enjoyable for others. They are ways to learn from each other. Ground yourself with your breathing. Be totally aware of what you want. If there's fear, why? What's at stake? Be totally aware of the other person's fear and what he or she wants. *Listen.* Repeat what you think you hear. *Clarify.* You don't have to agree, but hold yourself and others in high esteem. Be ready to compromise. Know where you have to draw the line to be true to yourself.

When you feel like climbing the walls, climb them. Do a Handstand, Half Headstand, or Half Shoulderstand against the wall. The Bottoms Up Configuration smooths out your worry lines . . . and your worries. Do them before an important meeting in which you want to be your very best. I know a top executive who does a Handstand before every board meeting and a Coffee Break Stretch before making any major decision. Others take their shot in the glass. He gets his from UEs.

Standitis

What is standitis? It's the pain in the feet, legs, and back that you get from standing . . . and standing . . . and standing. All of you who have to stand to work are likely to fall heir to this occupational hazard: teachers, nurses, doctors, technicians, dentists, traffic cops, clerks, chiefs, performers, and scores of other professionals.

You are fortunate if you can move around while you stand. But some people have to stand in one spot for hours. The first three configurations—One-Leggers, Angles, and Legs—are designed for curing standitis. You'll see how many wily little subterfuges you can do while standing on the job.

Mary Mulligan manages a Waldens book store in Denver. After raising five children, she's still on her feet all day in the book store.

Mary comes to class each week with her two daughters. Then at work she incorporates what she has learned in class. She uses a One-Step Backbend for reaching books on the tops shelves. As a runner and cyclist, she uses every chance she gets to stretch and twist on the job (Figure 6.4). She gets the whole staff going by making a game out of getting a job done. This book store is a fun place. It reflects her enthusiasm and energy. Mary says she's instinctively practiced UEs all her life to make her work easier: "I can't believe I've been doing UEs all this time!"

Here are some tips that will help you stand standing. Can you guess the first tip? You've got it! *Squirm!* If you need some lessons, watch children. They shift their weight, dance, shuffle, and squirm. The pain of standing is from standing still too long—and all wrong!

The second tip is your *posture picture.* No, this isn't going to be the same old stuff you heard day after day from your mother. "Pull your shoulders back, stand up straight!" That's too rigid and inflexible. Instead, enlist the support of your body. Use the arches of your feet and pelvic floor muscles.

The arches are the architectural wonders of your body. Imagine them like doorway arches supporting your body weight. Your pelvic floor muscles work in much the

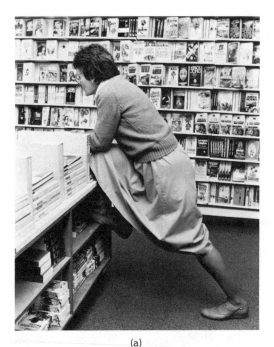

(a)

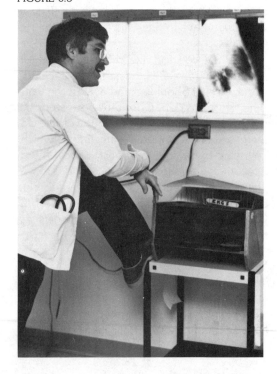

(b)

FIGURE 6.4

same way to support your abdominal organs. Use Pelvic Floor Pull-Ups and the lift of your arches to support and strengthen the foundation upon which you stand. Then hang in alignment.

Imagine that you are hanging from a sky hook. This will give you a beautiful, regal carriage. Not stiff and uptight, but light, free, and confident. Plant your feet, balance your pelvis, lift your sternum, relax your shoulders, center your head, and keep growing up.

UEs are so natural that instinctively you, like Mary Mulligan, use them to ease the strain of standing on the job. You find yourself propping your foot up on something . . . anything! It helps to lengthen your back and tuck your pelvis. This doctor (Figure 6.5) very casually does a Runner's Lunge as he examines x-rays. The stretching and breathing helps you stay focused on the job at hand whether it's a diagnosis, a sales pitch, or a lecture.

Dr. Jim Mosby, who wrote part of the

FIGURE 6.5

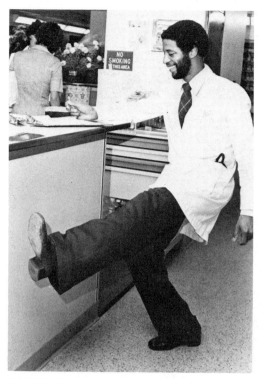

FIGURE 6.6

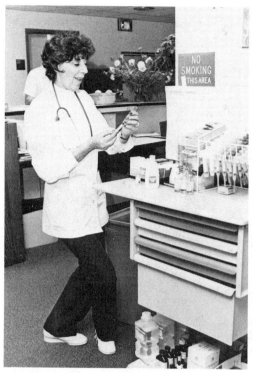

FIGURE 6.7

FIGURE 6.8

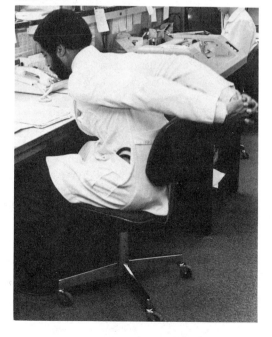

preface for this book, uses Hot Dog to take the fatigue out of his legs and back (Figure 6.6). A quick bend in one leg and kick up with the other helps you get a kick out of keeping records.

Use the UEs most helpful for the unique problems of your working situation. Use any chance you get to lean your back against a wall. It'll lengthen the lifespan of your back and legs. Mogul and Back Press are priceless friends on the job.

This nurse does Standing Eagle as she prepares medications (Figure 6.7). She injects humor and fun into the difficult task of helping people get well again.

Dr. Mosby does a Coffee Break Stretch as often as possible throughout the day or night (Figure 6.8). It clears the mind, sharpens the senses, and restores wit and humor during those long hours. He likes the Doorknob Squat too, or a Split-Leg Forward Bend. It

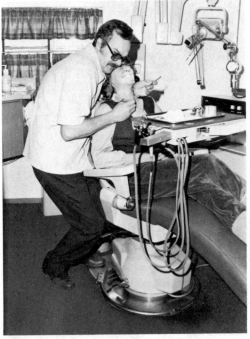

FIGURE 6.9

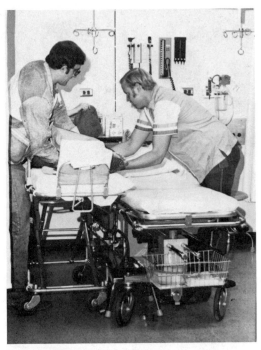

FIGURE 6.10

FIGURE 6.11

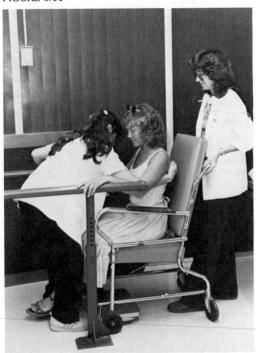

gets you breathing again and keeps your legs in shape.

Dentists have a back-breaking job leaning over mouths all day. Our dentist uses his great sense of humor to get you through the fear and discomfort of dental work. He often sits down on the job or works with one foot up on a prop (Figure 6.9).

Physical therapists, paramedics, and other medical personal often have to support, carry, or lift their patients. Use the fulcrum-lever concept to keep your back safe, as the pros do in Figure 6.10.

In Figure 6.11, a physical therapist aide is helping me get out of a wheelchair. Notice that she's lifting with her legs bent. She's also using her breath to give her the strength and energy to support additional weight. When you lift, *don't* hold your breath. *Exhale* and lift. Breathe rhythmically as you hold or carry the extra weight. Rely on your Core Power to support and sustain you. It will help you balance your pelvis and safeguard your spine.

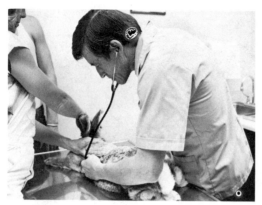

FIGURE 6.12

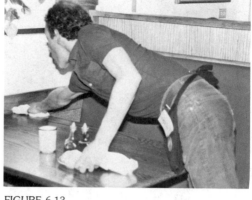

FIGURE 6.13

Our vet, Doc Sargent, has seen us through many emergencies and tough decisions with our pets. He bends over all day long as he examines little critters like Tibbar (Figure 6.12). He can take the strain off his back by doing Split-Leg Forward Bend or Standing Eagle. As a marathon runner, Doc Sargent can use these undercover stretches and strengtheners to his advantage.

Hairdressers and barbers have to stand all day, too, but they can do UEs to ease their backs and stay focused on their masterpieces. Balance the pelvis and relieve back strain by propping one foot up on a prop. Use a Split-Leg Forward Bend to stretch hamstrings while you do a shampoo.

Restaurant work is one of the most stressful professions. Waiters and waitresses are caught between the customer and the chef or the boss. Do UEs to calm and center yourself. They help maintain that positive, friendly attitude. Use Empathy Observation. Identify with what your boss wants and what the customer wants. You are often a peacemaker. Your job is providing a pleasant atmosphere and meal for each of your customers. It takes self-discipline and the ability to "cartoon it" when dealing with rudeness, pettiness, and especially those quarter tips!

Here's a great way to relieve stored tension and fatigue. This waiter is doing a Split-Leg Forward Bend while he clears his table (Figure 6.13). Throw in a twist now and then (Figure 6.14), and he has his winning edge over the afternoon.

When your back is "breaking," squat to pick up supplies. Remember to carry your trays with Core Power. Bend your knees slightly and use Hot Dog as you put down or carry food.

FIGURE 6.14

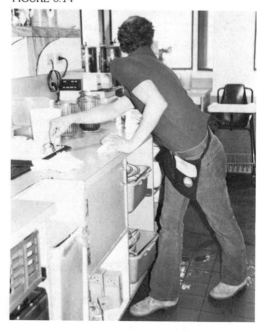

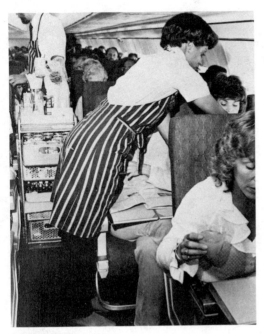

FIGURE 6.15

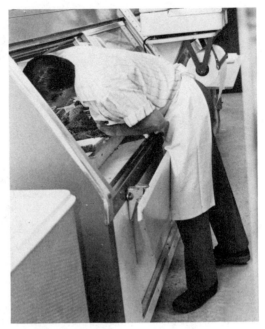

FIGURE 6.16

United Airline attendants get in some good UEs as they serve lunch (Figure 6.15). This attendant is using a 90° Forward Bend, but if you have a bad back, be sure to protect it with a Bent Leg or Split-Leg Forward Bend (see Chapter 3). Squatting down to get drinks is a great way to get in a workout on board. Every chance you get for a stretch helps you cope with the effects of air travel.

Grocers get their share of UEs. Figure 6.16 shows opportunity for a Split-Leg Forward Bend. This New York City vendor is doing a Bent-Knee Forward Bend (Figure 6.17). He's got lots of chances for UEs! Vendors lift and squat all day. Hamstring stretches with a One-Legger on a box can lessen the strain on your back and legs.

As this policeman listens to a tourist, he does a One-Legger (Figure 6.18). It's natural and feels good. UEs are the living strategies that bring life, energy, and calmness into what we do.

Just putting one leg on the step of this bus gives the policeman a much-needed rest

from pounding the pavement (Figure 6.19). Use your x-ray vision and notice how the pelvis is tucked and the lumbar curve lengthened by simply putting one leg up on the step.

Bending, Lifting, and Reaching on the Job
Landscapers, mechanics, carpenters, paint-

FIGURE 6.17

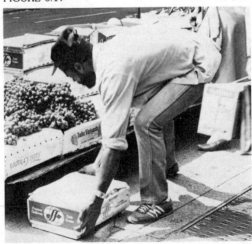

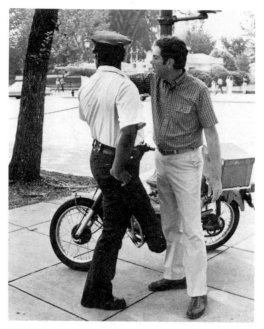

FIGURE 6.18

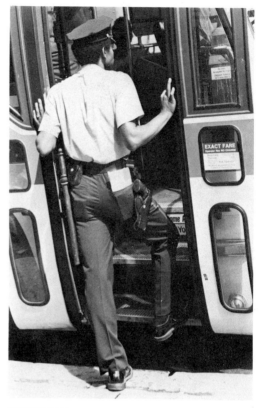

FIGURE 6.19

ers, construction workers, road crews, repair men and women, farmers, and ranchers have super workouts built right into their jobs.

Window washing isn't usually considered fun, but the gentlemen in Figure 6.20A–B go after it like true Undercover Agents. Figure 6.20A shows a Kneeling Squat. Notice the stretch for back and legs. The peace in this face reminds us that it's not *what* you do but *how* that makes the difference. Reaching out over a Split-Leg Forward Bend puts the Fulcrum-Lever Concept to work (Figure 6.20B). Desk workers may want to take time out to do a few windows!

Look at the workout this telephone repairman gets (Figure 6.21). Reaching and twisting to string new line, he's doing a great Dynamic Duo to hold his position. The toolbelt helps him tuck his pelvis. Breathing rhythmically can help him concentrate and stay alert, no matter what weather or working conditions impose on him.

All dock-workers, delivery people, movers, carriers, lifters and loaders—lift and

carry additional weight with your legs, abdominals, arm and chest muscles, *not* your back! Review the section in Chapter 3 on safe principles of lifting. Practice the Squat and Lunge Configurations. Do the Jumping Suns to keep your upper body strong and ready for lifting. Constantly practice Core Power exercises so that you can turn on that power when you need it. Use One-Legger and Runner's Lunge as often as you can to counteract the shortened muscles from the work.

When you lift, keep your knees bent. Juggle the extra weight as close to your body as possible. Hold your torso firmly in Cosmic Sandwich. You may need to keep your pelvis tucked rather than balanced as you lift and carry heavy loads. *Use your breath!* Inhale, get set. Exhale, lift. (See Figure 6.22.) As you lift and carry, use rhythmical breathing for

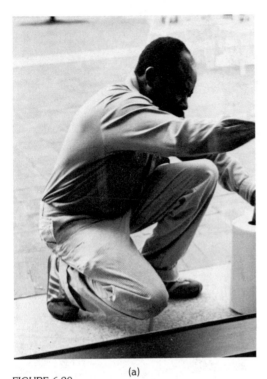

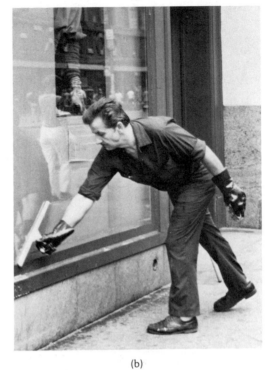

(a)   (b)

FIGURE 6.20

FIGURE 6.21   FIGURE 6.22

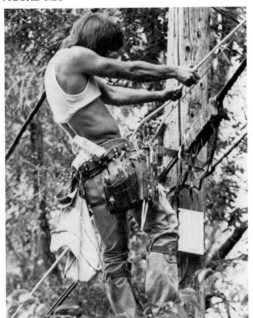

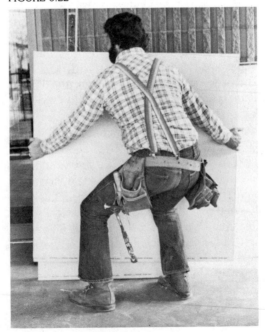

support. Use the support of your pelvic floor muscles and Core Power to sustain the weight of your load and to protect your back! Your training in Rhythmical Complete Breathing pays off here.

Working on cars is a livelihood for some and a hobby for others. Figure 6.23 shows how natural it is to tip into the See Saw from a 90° Forward Bend (chair workout under Sititis). Here the fulcrum happens to be the car fender rather than the back of a chair. Beware! Cars can eat you alive!

Figure 6.24 shows my son Jamie installing the rollbar he bought shortly after my accident. Good thing, too! A few months later, he rolled his truck on a mountain road and lived to tell about it. Notice the Bent Leg Forward Bend position that supports his back and reduces strain.

Construction work can be grueling and dangerous. The crew is always on the move, kneeling, bending, lifting, carrying, twisting, and turning (Figure 6.25). An Undercover Agent on a construction job has unlimited potential for weight training and UEs built right into the job. The worker in Figure 6.26 uses his whole body instead of straining his back to push his heavy machinery.

Jack hammers are like motorized bucking bronchos! Back-breaking work! The man in Figure 6.27 is trying to work in a backbreaking position. The strain to his lower back is enormous! A Split-Leg position would be much safer. *Bend the knees and use the Fulcrum-Lever Concept.*

Firemen are always ready to hop to it with One-Leggers, Runner's Lunges, Twists, Squats, and smiles (Figure 6.28). They really *do* come to your rescue. Thanks, guys!

Painting is a pain in the neck. One of the

FIGURE 6.23

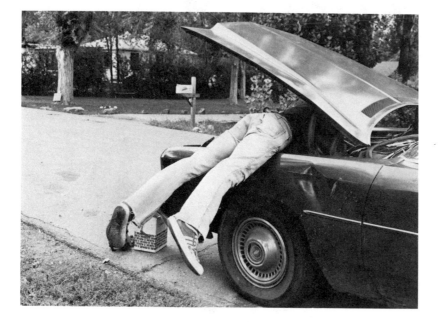

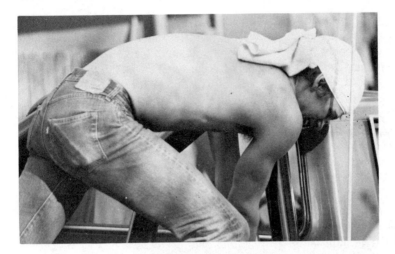

FIGURE 6.24

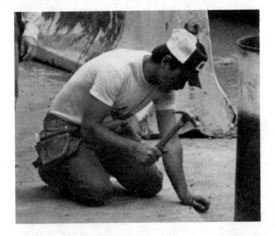

FIGURE 6.25

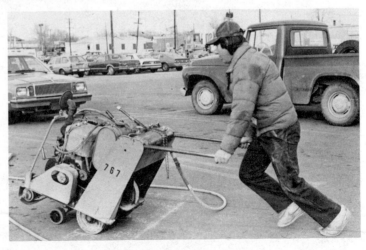

FIGURE 6.26

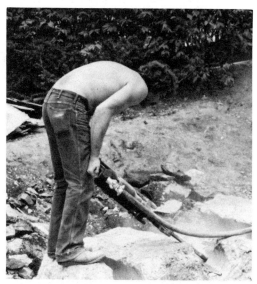

FIGURE 6.27

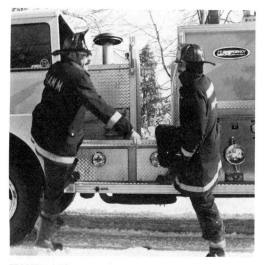

FIGURE 6.28

FIGURE 6.29

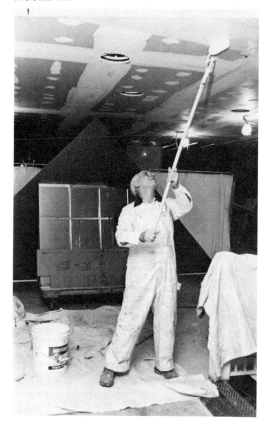

occupational hazards is compression of the neck and lower back. This gentleman (Figure 6.29) has had a lot of experience! He's learned from years of on-the-job training to incorporate Dynamic Duo to save his back and neck.

If you've ever tried to replace a drain-pipe under the sink you know what kind of exercise plumbers get! Kneeling Squats, twists and pretzellike configurations are the tricks of the trade. This plumber (Figure 6.30), gets his undercover workout digging sewer lines, un-clogging pipes, and so on. He and his wife run their own business. They don't have time for athletic clubs, but they find plenty of ways to work out on the job.

Figure 6.31 shows the "brain surgeon" who came to the rescue of our pet word pro-cessor, "E.T." Bending over like this all day can be a pain! Repairmen and women need to implement Bent-Leg Forward Bends, Split-Leg Forward Bends, and Hot Dogs into their work. Squats and Back Presses against a wall between jobs can also help tremen-dously.

This couple (Figure 6.32A—B) must do

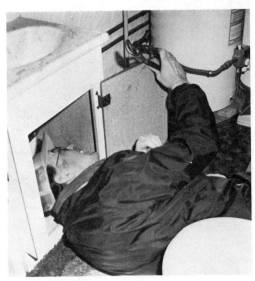

FIGURE 6.30

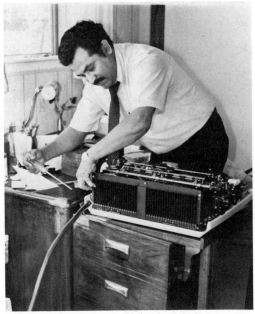

FIGURE 6.31

hundreds of Kneeling Squats, Split-Leg Forward Bends, and Flying One-Leggers before they're ready to start their fulltime jobs. They do their aerobic workout by walking briskly from door to door. They bend, stoop, and jump porch steps as they deliver papers to every door. Both walk to and from work every day. Why do they deliver newspapers? "It helps get the kids through school, gives us a good morning workout, and above all it's a chance for us to be together in a very special way."

THE PAUSE THAT REFRESHES

Sneaky Breaks

Take small sneaky breaks as you work. The head dietician at a hospital does One-Leggers while she talks on the phone. She mentioned that she had trouble with her hamstrings when she started aerobic dancing. After doing UEs throughout the day, those boinger hamstrings began to relax and

stretch. In a week she was noticing a big difference.

We get so compressed from daily pressures. We yield to the pull of gravity and let the loads we carry weigh us down. We stay in the same old slouch-and-grouch we've been in all day. When you find yourself in this shape, Configuration Slump, turn around with UEs. It's time for a breath and a stretch!

Change your position as often as possible. Be aware of every opportunity to sneak a stretch and breathe. All the UEs you learned to do at your desk can be your sneaky little breaks. Dolores optimizes a turn to speak to a client by pushing against the desk for a good twist (Figure 6.33). Sneaky, right? Little breaks like this keep you alert and perky.

Big Breaks

Big breaks are quickie workouts that give you a break. Do a series of Jumping Lunges at a wall, window, or desk. Take Runner's Lunge position. Place your hands on the edge of a sturdy table or desk. Then jump from one

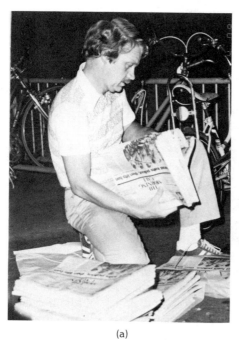

(a)

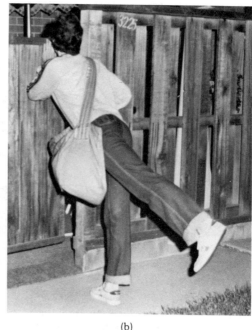

(b)

FIGURE 6.32

lunge into another (Figure 6.34) until you're ready to stop. This is an instant de-stressor.

If the Jumping Lunges are too much for you, do the Diamond Gait. Remember it? You were introduced to it in the lavatory of

FIGURE 6.33

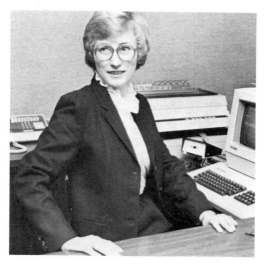

the airplane. It's a good mini-workout. It'll jog your brain into a calmer and clearer state.

Even when you go to the bathroom, UEs go with you! Use your foot to push the flush button on the wall—it's a dynamite One-Legger! Do a Hot Dog or Mogul if your back is sore and tired. If your knees can't take it, then lean up against the wall and do Wall Press, flattening your back to the wall.

The Suspension Bridge makes use of ledges everywhere. Use windowsills, desks, porches, or anything you can find to get in a good shoulder, arm, back, and leg stretch.

Get someone to take a break with you. My son Chris and his friend Roy are doing the Partner Tree Pose (Figure 6.35) during a study break. They'll be able to organize and store information much more effectively when they get through. You can read how to do the pose in Chapter 8.

Bus drivers have to sit for hours at a time. Figure 6.36 shows a bus driver moving luggage and getting in a UE at the same time.

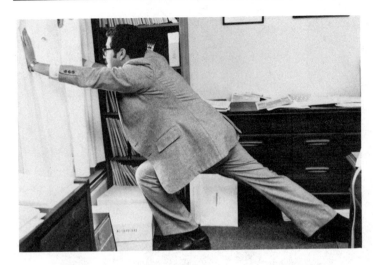

FIGURE 6.34

He's doing a Half Squat and getting back some life and energy.

Find some stairs for a good workout. Run up and down the stairs for a 15-minute aerobic workout, but be sure to train first. It's strenuous! Then do a series of Runner's Lunges to stretch your legs. Take three or four stairs at a time and stretch out your quads. Hold each stretch before going to the next stretch. Feels marvelous!

FIGURE 6.35

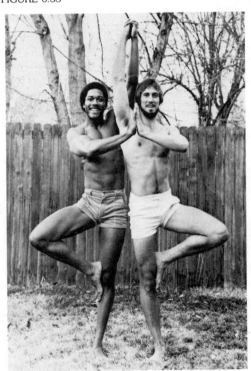

FIGURE 6.36

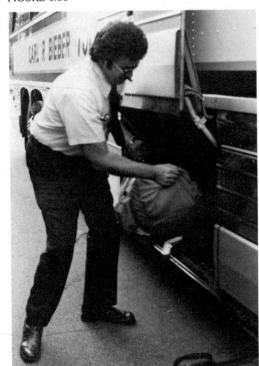

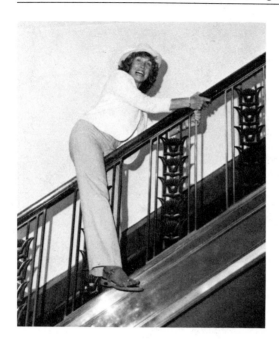

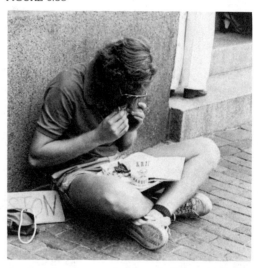

FIGURE 6.37

FIGURE 6.38

Finish off your staircase workout by . . . sliding down the banister (Figure 6.37)! It gets you in touch with that fun, exciting, childlike spirit again. It's a recharge!

Lunch breaks feed more than your stomach! They're food for your soul! Use all the tips in Chapter 7, Under the Tablecloth, to help you digest your meal. Don't overload, or your afternoon will be miserable. You'll just vegetate and get nothing, or very little, accomplished!

Eat your lunch outdoors or near a window. Let the outdoors refresh your spirits. If you've been sitting all morning, take a stand-up break for lunch. How about a slice of New York pizza? A lunchtime break can be wherever you are. In Figure 6.38 we caught a hitchhiker enroute sitting in Tailor Pose before he hits the road again.

Relaxation Breaks

Relaxation breaks can be as natural as getting a drink of water. They can be sneaky breaks, like a big yawn (Figure 6.39), or a stretch, or a

moment with your eyes closed. They can be a 1-minute part of a Big Break or your lunch break.

You have the tools and techniques to survive! You can shut it all off for a few moments and retreat to your power source, your center. You've practiced this in your Undercover Take-Off. Use any of the breathing exercises for 5 to 10 minutes. Then do Relaxation Pose in your chair (Figure 6.40A—B), on the floor, or in the park.

This is a retreat for recharging, a time for reflection. Use Empathy Observation as a way of clearing misunderstandings. Imagine that you are looking at yourself through another person's eyes. Notice how you look, act, and speak. Perhaps you'll understand something new about how others interpret your behavior. Seeing ourselves as others see us is a gift of perspective not often sought and less often perceived. When you feel neglected and unappreciated, cartoon it! See yourself in the funny papers.

Making the bridge from job to home

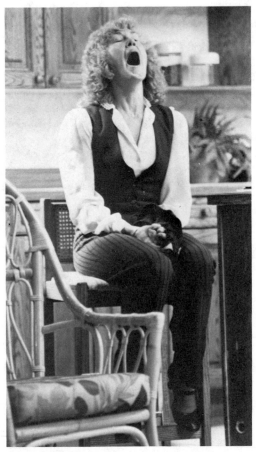

FIGURE 6.39

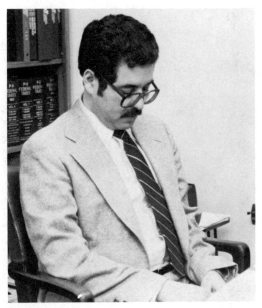

FIGURE 6.40 (a)

takes some deep breathing and debriefing. Review your day, your accomplishments, and what is left to be done. Leave your injuries and frustrations behind. That's easier said than done, but try! Debrief with a brisk walk, a run, or a few Sun Swings. Debrief your body *and* your mind. Don't go home without it!

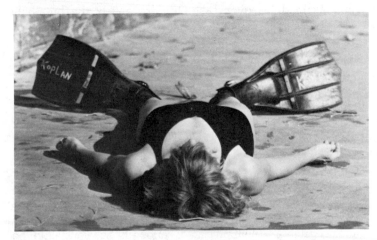

FIGURE 6.40 (b)

7

Under the Guise of the Mundane

Happiness is not doing what you like, but liking what you
have to do.

Well, we've all got it: the sameness of the nitty-gritty of daily living. We all have certain chores to do in order to live. It can get pretty old, pretty fast! "Everdayism" is a disease that eats away at projects, marriages, romances, jobs, material possessions, and our self-concepts. It takes a lot of heart, creativity, energy, and consistent, persistent work to keep a relationship or an enterprise alive and growing. It's a "soul-stretching convenant," as my Dad always says, "with the emphasis on stretching!"

An Undercover Agent is an alchemist, transforming the common and ordinary into something of promise and value. You have to be able to make something out of nothing. That was my mother's speciality. She taught us how to make stone soup. Do you know the fable? Two soldiers came into a village cold and hungry. They conned the villagers into making a "magicial" soup. "All you need is a stone and a fire under a pot of water," they promised. As the stone simmered away over the fire, they suggested adding whatever the

villagers had on hand—a carrot, a head of cabbage, an onion, a potato or two, a rutabaga, a little salt, and a pinch of herbs. Voilà! Soup of the homemade kind.

There's magic in that! The magic is in using whatever you've got to create what you need. This chapter deals with how to do just that! Undercover Exercises inject humor and energy into everything you do. They will take you through your shopping, errands, house and garden work, and the daily art of dining and entertainment. UEs turn the disease of everydayism into a revolutionary way of living. It's very simple. Come on along and let's do it together!

THE SPORT OF SHOPPING

Some of us love it, some of us hate it, but almost all of us have to do it! We have to shop for our homes, our business, and our personal lives. We use it, run out of it and then go and get it again. But shopping needn't be a chore or a bore.

We need food every day, so groceries are a must. Your grocery cart can become a jungle gym as you wheel around the shop getting supplies. Dull routine becomes playground fun!

The Runner's Lunge is a gem. You can ease your back with one foot on the bottom rung of the cart. Now push the cart ahead of you and stretch into the lunge. Great stretch for your hip flexors! Helps you keep your pelvis balanced. Now stretch the forward leg out straight. Don't become a split personality over it (Figure 7.1).

Keep one foot propped up on the bottom rung of your cart while you reach for something on the top shelf or read labels to check ingredients. It will help you stay in a tucked pelvis position and lengthen your back.

When you bend over into the freezer or dairy case, don't round your back. This straight-legged, rounded-back position, shown in Figure 7.2A, will reward you with a backache! Do a Split-Leg Forward Bend instead, supporting your body weight on the rim of the case (Figure 7.2B). You can easily go one step farther and do a Flying One-Legger. Watch other shoppers. Some people

do it naturally. It feels good. All you have to do is make it a conscious UE.

Take a moment for Suspension Bridge while you wait your turn at the deli counter. Sure, it's okay. No one's looking. And if they are, smile; you're on Candid Camera!

Carry your groceries in a cart, not your arms. Unless you have very strong abdominals and legs, you're going to end up overloading your back.

Find interesting places to shop. The Village Roaster is an olfactory delight! Coffee beans are roasted right in the shop. What a wonderful potpourri of teas, spices, coffee, and luscious chocolates—an oasis of excellence in a desert of mediocrity. I always have to inspect what's new in cookware (Figure 7.3). Great chance to get in a Split-Leg Forward Bend! If you do a 90° Forward Bend to get to the bottom shelf, you've got to practice it every day in your Winning-Edge Workout. You can strain your back if you haven't practiced the Fulcrum-Lever Concept (Chapter 3). For reaching, use Dynamic Duo to elongate your spine in a One-Step Backbend. Get a good spinal stretch. Press your hand to your sacrum to help you tuck your pelvis (Figure 7.4).

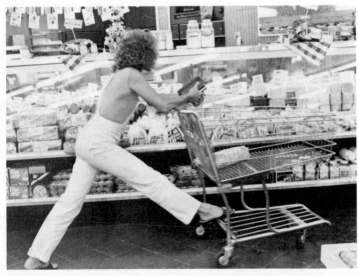

FIGURE 7.1

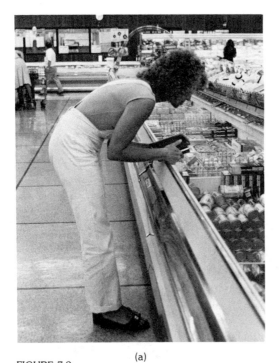
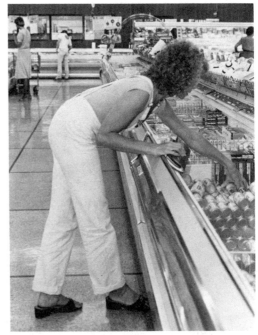

| (a) | (b) |

FIGURE 7.2

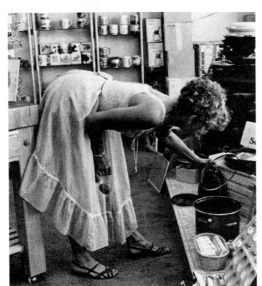

FIGURE 7.3

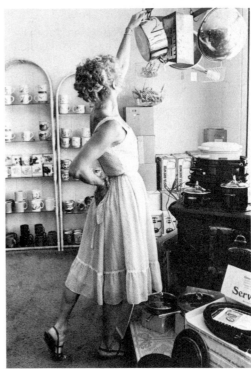

FIGURE 7.4

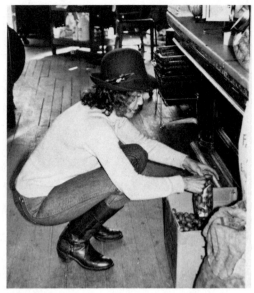

FIGURE 7.5

There's an old country store in Carbondale, Colorado, that has an old marble-topped counter for Suspension Bridge, barrels for One-Leggers, and even an old door for a Doorknob Squat. You can use a squat to stock up on chestnuts (Figure 7.5). It takes the strain out of your back from all the stop-and-go movements. Have you ever considered the miles you can rack up while shopping?

Running around from shop to shop is tiring. Wherever you find stairs, take time to do a Runner's Lunge. It's a natural way to work out those grumpies . . . and all undercover!

What kind of UEs can you do while shopping for clothes? This is the most tiring shopping of all! Put it on, take it off, put it on, take it off. It's not unusual to find me in a corner somewhere or between the clothes racks doing a One-Legger or a Coffee Break Stretch with a Forward Bend. I find getting blood to my brain essential for all those decisions!

As you can see in Figure 7.6, stools and counters are also good places for UEs. A Head Roll-Up for your abdominal's or Relaxa-

tion Pose right here? Why not? Get your feet up and stretch out.

Make-up counters can help you do the best you can with the best that you've got! View the raw material. Have fun dressing it up! Lean forward, resting your arms on the counter (Figure 7.7). Your legs can be in Suspension Bridge, Split-Leg Forward Bend, or Standing Eagle.

Escalators, stairs, and elevators are the spice of the shopper's life. Bar Swings on the escalator make you feel young and carefree again, but don't try them if you haven't done your homework. You need to train your arms, chest, and shoulder muscles to lift your torso, and your abdominals and thighs to lift your legs. Practice Bar Hangs and Sun Power in your Winning-Edge Workout before you attempt this. If the escalator swing isn't your style, just do a One-Legger with one foot on the handrail or one foot on the stair above

FIGURE 7.6

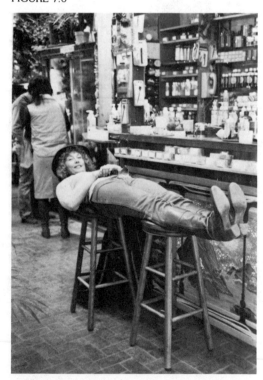

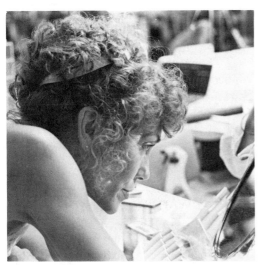

FIGURE 7.7

you. You can do Runner's Lunge on the escalator just as you did on the stairs (see Chapter 6).

Every water fountain offers a chance for a One-Legger and fluid replacement (Figure 7.8). Both are of vital importance for your energy level.

Elevators! The old kind with a walking, talking operator can make your day. Isn't it interesting to be in a crowded elevator so intimately involved with strangers that you can smell their cologne, hair spray, or coffee breath? It's amazing how we end up squooshed between perfectly strange bodies. How do you respond to becoming a sardine? Panic, dislike, disgust? Or can you for a few moments try Empathy Observation and be with the mass or energy that is part of you? Lucky you if you get an empty elevator! Do a few UEs before you get to the next stop.

Revolving doors are like carousels. But don't forget to get off! Take a few whirls (Figure 7.9) and get rid of your blahs.

Think of that check-in phone call as a chance to rejuvenate. Telephone booths are great places for doing UEs. Turn Configuration Slump (Figure 7.10A), which cuts off

your resources, into Staff Pose and practice Cosmic Sandwich (Figure 7.10B). Let your breathing be full and rhythmical. Count your breaths as you center yourself. You're more able to focus on the person you're calling.

If the conversation goes on and on, stretch one leg up in a hamstring stretch (Figure 7.11). Think of all the fun things you can do in the One-Legger configuration. Implement a stretch of your own. You can twist, turn, or even backbend in the phone booth.

Breaks are very important if you expect to survive shopping with any kind of aplomb. UEs on escalators and stairs are on-the-go breaks, but you need to take a Big Break in the lounge or on a bench. Undercover, do the tense-release exercise. Sometimes we need to create more tension to release tension. *Contract* your muscles—thighs, arms, chest, shoulders, jaws. Hold it! Now release and relax. Do this several times. Feel the energy re-

FIGURE 7.8

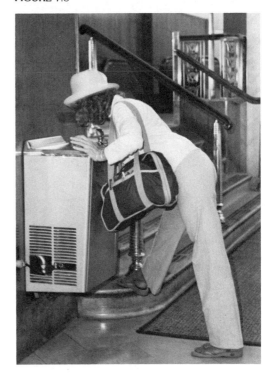

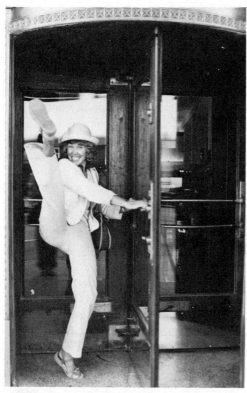

FIGURE 7.9

placing your tension. Turn your tension into a free-flowing energy that will revive and invigorate you.

Then with your eyes open practice the counting breaths, Chapter 2, or Relaxation Pose. Going inside while you are totally present outside is practicing consciousness on all levels at once. Practice that art in busy, noisy places. It prepares you for the situations that demand your total awareness.

WAITING IN LINES

Hurry up and wait! Is there anything more frustrating than a long line on top of a deadline? Have you ever noticed the faces of people waiting in lines? A recent visitor from East Germany was surprised at how easy shopping is for Americans. That certainly wasn't my view until she told us about the lines she stands in to get the simplest of life's necessities. So let's count our blessings and look like we've been blessed! Do UEs in line to ease tension and frustration. Once you've

FIGURE 7.10

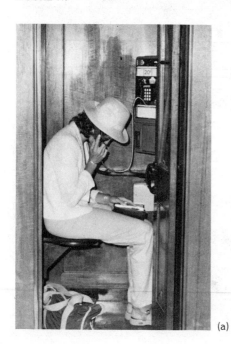

(a)

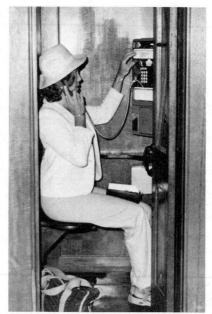

(b)

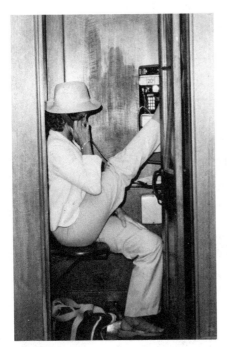

FIGURE 7.11

strengthen your legs (Figure 7.13). Our good friend Bob Moore has seen us through many packages. He's used to watching me sink out of sight! If you don't like such overt UEs, do Mountain Pose. Train yourself to stand with lightness anytime, anywhere, under any circumstance. It puts you at ease in the tensest situations and promotes a sense of strength and elegance.

FIGURE 7.12

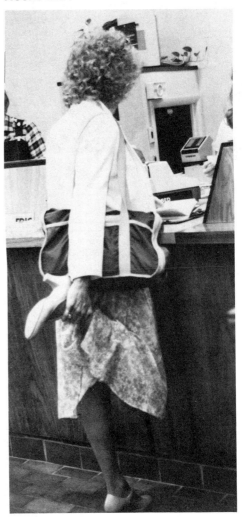

caught on to the idea of squirming, you'll come up with some of your own UEs. These are some of the standards. While you balance your checkbook at the bank, balance your body in Standing Eagle. Once you get to the teller's window you can do Standing Bow (Figure 7.12). That stretches your thighs after the work in Standing Eagle. If you don't feel comfortable grasping your ankle, don't! Just bend your knee to a 90° position and hold it level with your other knee.

A student told me that she had always despised errands. They made her absolutely frantic. A go-fers job is a hassle! Now she challenges herself to see how many UEs she can do while going-for-it. Her dreaded errands are more fun.

Standing in line at the post office can be an energizing, rather than exasperating, experience. You can do a One-Legger while waiting for your turn or do as the kids do . . . squirm. Dance a little, shift your weight, move. While your packages are weighed, do Hot Dog to

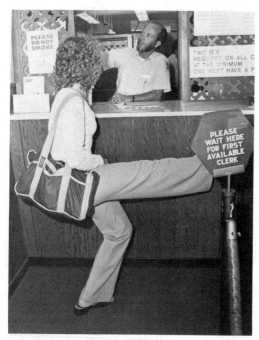

FIGURE 7.13

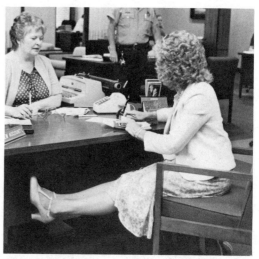

FIGURE 7.14

APPOINTMENTS

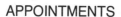

While you wait for appointments, do some subtle twists in the chair with your legs crossed or parallel to each other. Breathe smoothly as you go into the twist. The rhythmical breathing and twisting keep you calm. Practice your Pelvic Floor Pull-Ups. No one will know you're practicing your secret UEs, and they'll be helping to take the nervous jitters out of waiting.

Figure 7.14 proves that there are ways of working out while you talk to a bank officer, insurance agent, lawyer, or doctor. Do Double Leg or Knee Lifts. They give you the stomach for your banking transactions, insurance claims, or diagnosis.

At the beauty salon you can really let down your hair while you wait. Do your body a favor while your hair gets one. Work out a little and emerge a total make-over! It'll cost the same and you'll get a lot more for your money. Beautiful hair, beautiful body. As you enjoy your shampoo, get your feet up. Sit in Tailor Pose or Huggy Pose with your spine straight (Figure 7.15).

Get your feet up on the rung of the

FIGURE 7.15

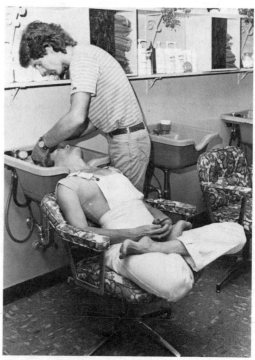

chair. Do a Knee-to-Chest Squeeze (Figure 7.16). That'll help elongate your back and relieve tension in your lower back and hips.

You can get in an abdominal workout with Double or Single Leg or Knee Lifts. Hide it all under the smock. Tom is an understanding hairdresser. He doesn't mind a few UEs. The results complement his efforts!

OPERATION HOME BASE

Home is your castle, your fortress away from the hustle and bustle, a place where you can be yourself. What you are at home reflects how you feel about yourself and your relationships with those closest to you. It's easier to be fun and entertaining out there on the job than it is when the draperies are drawn, the bills need paying, and the kids are arguing.

Love makes the world go round and turns a house into a home. It creates a loving community of trust and loyalty in which we can learn to be our best selves, a place where we can be vulnerable and self-revealing without fear of ridicule. Some people have a gift for making an acquaintance feel like a long-time friend. But as Richard Restak says in *The Self Seekers*, if you treat long-time friends as if they are acquaintances, then you are unable to reveal your idiosyncracies in a long-term, in-depth relationship. We don't want to live in a family of acquaintances, but a fellowship of friends. A friend is someone who helps us be more ourselves.

The family in America is in jeopardy. It is suffering the growth pains of change, but it must still be the center of where we mature, where we nuture and support each other. Whether it is a group of people connected by blood lines or a group of people chosen to be family to each other, this unit is the foundation of relationships.

In stress-management seminars run by Humanics Co., we have found that people are primarily interested in resolving their

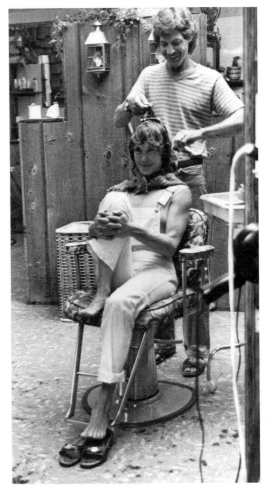

FIGURE 7.16

interpersonal conflicts at home. Job-related problems take second place to problems with family and friends. In fact, it's usually the home conflicts or other non-job-related conflicts that instigate the problems at work. How many of you have had a terrible day at the office because you had a bad morning at home?

Creating a harmonious living place and space for all family members is an endeavor that demands the greatest self-discipline, self-sacrifice, and teamwork. It's a tough job, and the rewards don't include awards, laurels, medals, raises, letters of appreciation, or public accolades. Anyone who has raised a family knows you gotta have a lot of heart. We sustain, support, and stand by each other (Figure 7.17). Families give us the time and space to grow and sort it all out, to learn about personal responsibility and the cause and effects of what we think, say, and do.

If we play together, we'll stay together. Our pets and our friends teach us responsibility (Figure 7.18). Undercover Exercise can help us be together in different ways that expand our awareness and appreciation of each other. UEs cross age and communication barriers. Playing and working together in new ways reduce the stresses and strains that weaken and sometimes fracture the family unit.

FIGURE 7.17

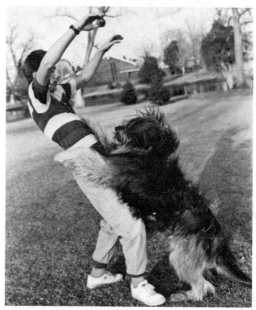

FIGURE 7.18

Set aside regular daily or weekly times to be together doing chores or a special project. Make it fun, a game, a contest. Make a contract with yourself and the others. Agree on what you want to accomplish and how long it will take, and then go for it 100 percent!

Sometimes jobs are disagreeable and hard. I remember one project of cutting down and hauling thorny bushes. Ugh! Singing songs to get through it, the thorns didn't seem so bad.

Health Club in The Garden

Under the guise of gardening is a potential workout that not even a health club can touch! It all depends on how you do it. Approach your gardening as you would an active meditation. It's like a run, a game of tennis, a swim. Focus on the sights, sounds, smells, and textures of the garden. Think about the seeds that will germinate in the earth or the coming harvest. Then focus on how many UEs you can do while you workplay! Here are a few to get you started.

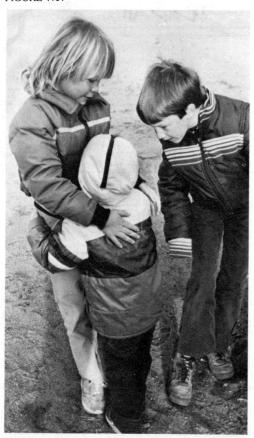

Weeding is one of my favorite meditations. I think of how my grandmother dug sandspurs on her hands and knees so the children could walk barefoot in the grass. I'm reminded of all the junk I'd like to weed out of my life and my thoughts. It's weeding-out therapy for me. Don't get caught up in over-reaching. You'll pay for it when you try to get out of bed the next morning! Use the Squat for awhile. Change to the Split-Leg Forward Bend for the next patch of weeds. Leaning on your forward leg helps you support your back (Figure 7.19). It's a nice resting pose. Honest! Alternating between these UEs gives your legs a workout and interesting ways to cover a lot of ground.

Reaping the harvest is a mixed blessing. Gathering enough for a big rhubarb pie means washing and preparing it too. I used to spend hours at the kitchen sink washing veggies until I realized that I didn't *have* to stand the backache. I got back to the basics with the Squat. I use the garden hose and I can work my legs while resting my back. It's a great way to wash veggies and water the lawn too! It's even a handy UE for winding the hose. You can go from a Half Squat to a Full Squat, from a 90° Forward Bend into Intense Forward Bend with bent knees. Wow! Does that work the legs . . . and save the back!

My husband's pride and joy is the garden. He does it all by hand so he can get in lots of UEs and lots of benefits. Since he refused to be photographed, Figure 7.20 shows *me* plowing our garden. This is a good time for Runner's Lunge.

If you've ever hoed potatoes or onions, you know what hard, back-breaking work it is. Change your position as often as you can. Alternate hoeing with other jobs. Keep your back straight and well supported.

When your back gets tired, hang out on a gate. Bend your knees and tuck your pelvis going down in a Half Squat or Full Squat. Stretch your back and hang in traction (Figure 7.21).

FIGURE 7.19

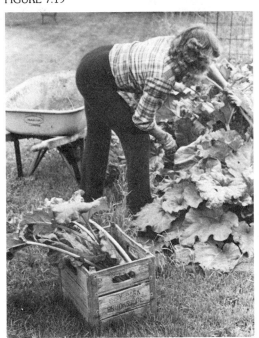

FIGURE 7.20

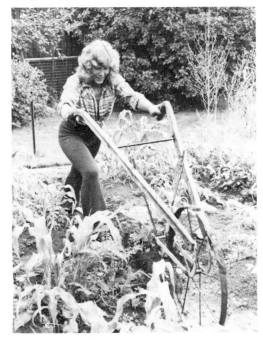

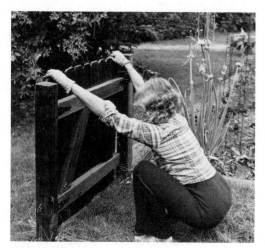

FIGURE 7.21

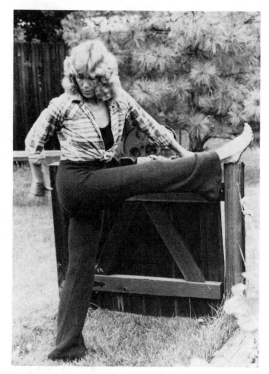

FIGURE 7.22

Then change the type of work again. How about loading the wheelbarrow? When you wheel a heavy load, keep your knees bent and your pelvis tucked in Half Squat. Use all the principles of safe lifting you learned in Chapter 3.

When you're lifting or carrying, juggle the weight until you can use your legs to support it. Hug it when you lift it! Move your load as close to your body as possible. Use your legs and abdominal muscles to lift, carry, or move the additional weight.

Stretch out your legs and back with a One-Legger Twist on a gate (Figure 7.22). Notice that this gate has no fence? I keep it to remind me of life's paradoxes! These sneaky breaks are vital. De-stressing the stressed parts of your body will keep you going and reduce fatigue.

Sit down on the job whenever you can. Gardening can cause stiffness and pain for days unless you learn how to wheel and deal with your joints. This is especially true for people with back and knee problems.

I'll share my secret garden magic with you: a rod or bar, two pieces of strong rope, and you've got a swing! (It also helps to have a tree.) Hang in traction with Bar Hangs or Hanging Bow and let your back lengthen with gravity (Figure 7.23). I couldn't garden without it! But sometimes you have to fight the kids to get a turn (Figure 7.24).

Celebrate the garden work! Picnic in the corn patch with wine, cheese, fresh veggies, and your favorite bread or crackers. Do some partner stretches together in the shade (Chapter 8). They finish off your garden workout and make you feel good.

There are always weeds to pull and leaves to rake. Garden work can sometimes feel endless, relentless, and fruitless. Our persistent, consistent work doesn't always pay off the way we think it should. In seconds, a hailstorm can leave our garden in shreds. Then what is left? What we've learned in the tilling. We may or may not enjoy the fruits of our labor. Farmers know that. But if we plant our apple tree today, we've done the best that we can with the best that we have, to be the best that we are.

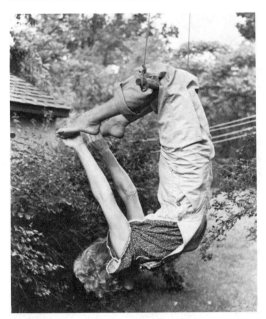

FIGURE 7.23

FIGURE 7.24

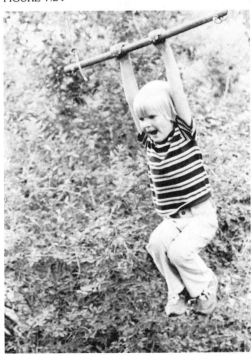

The House Spa

You've spent an hour cleaning the floors and shampooing the carpet. Before you know it, someone has tracked mud all over the house! Was it the dog, the kids, or the repairman? You're furious! Or you've just spent hours preparing a beautiful dinner, setting the table, and getting everyone together. It's been fun! But in less than an hour, the meal's over and there are dishes to do. And nobody really wants to do them! Is it worth it?

I don't think there's anything more repetitious, discouraging, and lonely than housekeeping and meal preparation. I'm not talking about the once-in-a-while gourmet dinner or the spring cleaning. I'm talking about the day-after-day cleaning, cooking, and upkeep of the house. This is what should win medals for bravery! It's hard, and the work never ends.

Here you are, faced with cooking and cleaning daily. What are you going to do with it? This chapter may be the best present you can give yourself . . . and your family or roommates. The first benefit is that UEs dilute negative self-pity when you're feeling stuck with all the work. And that's because the second benefit is to your body, the house that lives in your house.

Prioritize and systematize the jobs you want to get done. Be reasonable about what you can *get* done. Don't intimidate yourself. Then do your tasks in order of priority. Get the bread going first. As it raises, throw in the laundry. As it's swooshing, do the dusting, and so on. Invent a UE for *every* job you do. Think of the incredible workout you'll get. Picture yourself emerging from your house spa at the end of your day svelte, fascinating, and glamorous.

Cooking Hash or beans by candlelight can be a king's delight! There is no substitute for excellent food. But your delivery service can make the difference between common, ordinary grub and extraordinary culinary delights!

Here are some UEs that will take strain out of cooking and give you zest and energy for the delivery.

The kitchen is where this book was born. The yoga postures were fun to incorporate and helped relieve my back pain. I had to tuck my pelvis while reaching and lifting or I got "lumbar crunch" for lunch. As I bent down for a bowl, Split-Leg Forward Bend fell into place. After a few Standing Eagles, Hot Dogs, and twists, the kitchen work turned into an exhilarating workout.

Rule 1. Never Stand When You Can Sit. Get a high stool that you can move to the sink or chopping block. Sit while you do jobs that involve chopping, cleaning, and mixing.

Rule 2. Do UEs While You Work. Prop your foot on something for One-Legger (Figure 7.25). While you're standing, alternate between Tree, Standing Bow, and Standing Eagle. Remember to change legs and repeat the UE on the opposite side. When you have to reach for a bowl on the top shelf, use the One-Step Backbend. As you bend down for a pot in the cupboard, do a Squat or a Split-Leg Forward Bend (Figure 7.26).

FIGURE 7.26

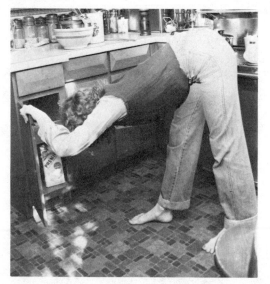

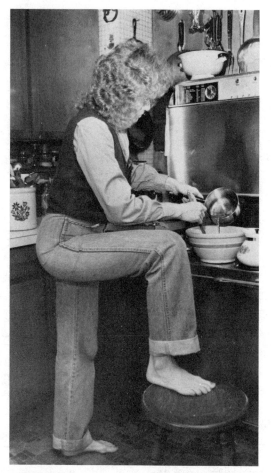

FIGURE 7.25

Rule 3. Take the Weight Off Your Back. Lean on a counter (Figure 7.27). The counter can help you support your body weight.

Food preparation can be a beautiful meditation. When you find yourself grumbling and grumping about what you're doing, focus on the aroma and texture and goodness of the ingredients. Let your outgoing breath be a thank-you for the food on your table. The breath of thankfulness turns a grump into a grateful cook!

All of us have to work around our limitations. My dad has a congenital malformation of the hip socket that has caused him pain since childhood. Its crippling effects would

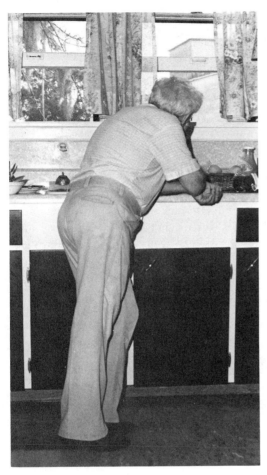

FIGURE 7.27

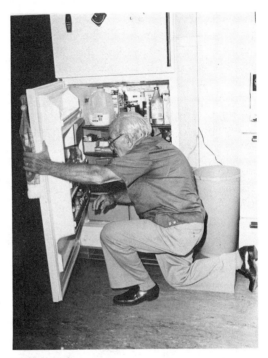

FIGURE 7.28

FIGURE 7.29

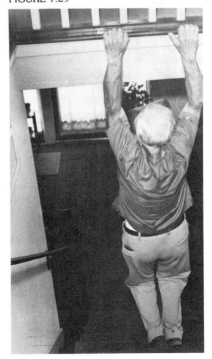

have slowed him down by now if he hadn't worked so hard at standing, walking, and moving in alignment. Dad has taught me a lot about pain, self-discipline, and the importance of alignment in our lives. He uses a Kneeling Squat (Figure 7.28) to get ingredients for his soup of the day. He makes frequent use of the Runner's Lunge, too, because of his bad hip. In his mid-seventies, he runs circles around men half his age! On top of his daily rounds at the hospital, he mows lawns, cooks for the senior guests at the lodge, digs septic tanks, and carries in the laundry. Every morning Dad lengthens his back by hanging from the stairwell (Figure 7.29). He does a few chin-ups before heading out. Simple UEs like these make all the difference in our lives. They take less time than it takes to pop a pill. Pop a UE or a pill. Which will you take?

Cleaning   Dreaded chores? Vacuuming and sweeping can be done aerobically to music. Put on your favorite album or, better yet, *sing* as you vacuum. You sound terrific over the noise of the machine, just as you do in the shower. There's a bonus in singing. It oxygenates your system and works your abdominals just like laughing. It also gives you a chance to air out your mouth! So belt out the tunes as you lunge and stretch, squat and lift. Support your weight whenever you can by holding on to a prop. It helps reduce back fatigue and reminds you to stay in alignment (Figure 7.30A). Glide into a Runner's Lunge (Figure 7.30B). Go for that long stretch in your thighs. Feel the wonderful release of tension in your back and legs.

Use the Squat to help you move furniture or lift that heavy plant or sculpture (Figure 7.31). The One-Step Backbend helps you reach to dust a shelf or get those cobwebs (Figure 7.32).

Telephone interruptions can be times for a break. Two good UEs for telephone breaks are the Standing Eagle and Tree Pose. If I get stuck on the phone I sit on the floor and do Sitting Eagle.

Take time for a quiet break. Go out under the trees and sit quietly (Figure 7.33). Tune into your breathing, go inside and reestablish your connection with your center.

FIGURE 7.30

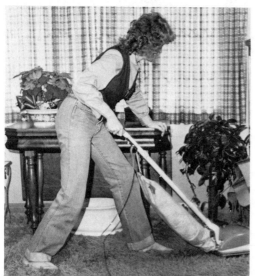

(a)

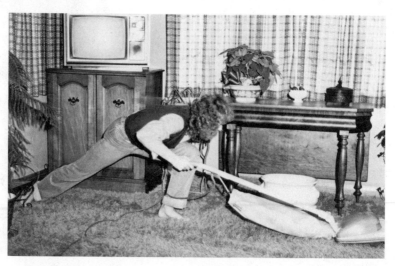

(b)

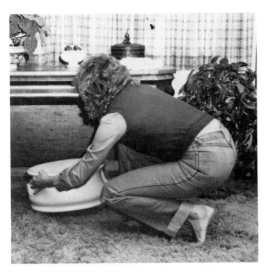

FIGURE 7.31

FIGURE 7.32

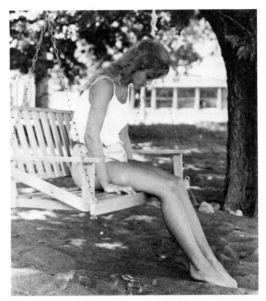

FIGURE 7.33

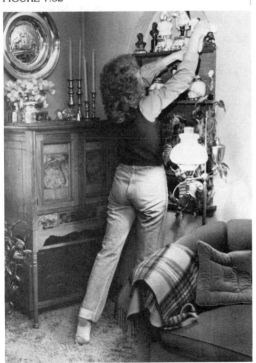

Finish off with a bath and UEs in the tub (see Chapter 8). You'll look and feel terrific for that night on the town . . . or around the dinner table.

What's it all for? Here's my pay-off for a long day of baking, cleaning, and gardening. I've had a great workout. In my heart I know I've done my best. The house is filled with the aroma of freshly baked bread. Friends and family take their places with anticipation. We smile as the hot loaves are passed around, each of us pulling off a piece of hot, steaming bread. In the glow of candles we say thanks. Adding butter, cheese, or marmalade, we feast like kings and queens! Our lives are lifted above the mundane as we share homemade bread around the family table.

UNDER THE TABLECLOTH

Now both of your houses are bright and shiny—your body-house and your house-house. You've had your workout at the spa.

Diets are a phenomenon born of affluence. We have the dubious distinction of being one of the few countries in the world that chooses to diet; most "dieters" in other cultures just cannot get enough food to eat.

If you practice your daily Winning-Edge Workout, sneak in UEs throughout the day, and choose wholesome foods to eat, dieting can be a fast of the past. The three essentials—circulation, alignment, and extension—will help you maintain your proper weight. Your proper weight is the weight at which you feel, look, and perform best. You and your doctor can determine that. Your fantasy of how you should look may not concur with your optimal weight. Many people suffer needless agony over trying to look like something their bodies cannot safely be.

Let's take the first of the three essentials, circulation. *Increase it!* Make a daily habit of spending as much time increasing your circulation as you do eating. No, it's not likely to increase your appetite. In fact, it'll do just the opposite. Research is showing that exercise decreases the appetite. Face-stuffing is usually not the result of hunger; its number-one cause is loneliness, boredom, and frustration!

Try this experiment. Stand in front of the open refrigerator. Looking for something? Before you raid it, do these three UEs. In Split-Leg Forward Bend, breathe three full breaths. Change legs and breathe three more. Keep looking. Then do a 90° Forward Bend. Hold on to the refrigerator and keep your back as straight as you can. Take three full breaths. Last but not least, do Flying One-Legger. Keep looking for something to nosh on! Hold on and lift one leg back behind you. Breathe three full breaths. Change legs and repeat. Now, are you still "hungry"? If yes, gleefully eat whatever you choose. Observe how you feel after eating. *Did you find what you were looking for?*

These three UEs will calm and reassure you and give you time to ask, "Am I really hungry? What do I really want?"

Now consider the second of the three

essentials, alignment. Working on your alignment in your daily Winning-Edge Workout teaches you to be aware of yourself, how your body feels, and the subtleties that affect it. Your workout makes you aware of and teaches you the consequences of excess. Balance and harmony begin to feel so good that you don't want to upset it. Sneaking in your UEs throughout the day and evening helps you stay centered and balanced. When you do binge or gorge, you pay. It doesn't feel good.

The last of the three essentials is extension. When you feel the lightness and ease of movement from doing UEs, it gets harder and harder to tolerate anything that denies you that feeling. Sometimes disappointment, grief, or anger upsets you, so you give up on your workout and pig out! That heavy, yucky feeling depresses you even more. It's back to the Winning-Edge Workout and UEs. They're still there! Voilà! You feel light and free and *good* again. You vow never to do it again, but of course you do. That's okay. You've got your survival tools. UEs are only a breath and a stretch away! Count on them!

Meal times are celebrations. *How* we eat is just as important as *what* we eat.

Whether you're dining out or at home, take a moment for quiet centering that can relax and prepare your digestive system for the intake of food. One of the most stressful things you can do is eat when you're upset. Negative thoughts and petty attitudes create indigestion. Unwind for a moment, say a quiet thank-you, and allow yourself to be sensitive to the joy of mealtime.

Here's how you do that. Sit in Staff Pose in your chair. You can keep your legs parallel or cross them unobtrusively in Tailor Pose under the table cloth, balancing your pelvis and lengthening your spine. This position allows plenty of room for the digestive organs to do their job without being all scrunched from slumping.

With your eyes open or closed, take at

least three to five rhythmical breaths. Do the Abdominal Breathing or Rhythmical Complete Breathing you practiced in your Undercover Take-off. Run a tension check all over your body. Do the tense-release technique you used in Chapter 7. Concentrate on tensing your legs, buttocks, abdomen, chest, and arms (under the table cloth). Then release. Breathe fully and express gratefulness in your own style. Now you're ready for a tasty meal.

If you happen to find yourself in a competitive or conflict situation with someone at the dining table, you can do two things. Eat lightly and only those foods you know you can digest easily. The other option is to remove yourself from the conflict with a Love Missile or Empathy Observation (Chapters 2 and 6). Let go of what you wish the other person would do to resolve the conflict.

Establishing mealtime traditions and rituals lends stability and regularity to our lives. But rituals can also turn into rigidity. You have to change now and then. Do the unaccustomed, the unexpected. Eat lunch on the roof. Have pizza for breakfast! Sing together. It's a great way to breathe together and dissolve tensions.

Eating can be an active meditation. Focus on the aroma, texture, color and taste of your food. Chew each bit thoroughly. Put down your spoon or fork after each bite. Only when your mouth is empty take another bite. Just like your breathing exercises—when your lungs are empty, you take in another breath. Notice how often you are eating mindlessly, just stuffing yourself. Eat and drink with total awareness. Honestly, you'll never have to worry about overeating! You'll be satisfied from head to toe. Each bite will be a meal in itself. "Why spend your money on what is not food and your earnings on what never satisfies?" Isaiah 55:2.

UEs before and after dinner can be artfully accomplished. Some of our students report that since they've started implementing UEs under the table cloth, their dispositions

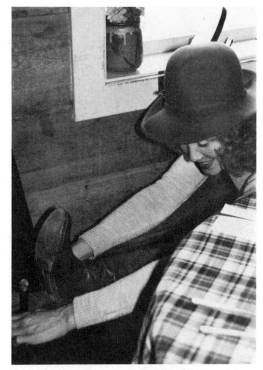

FIGURE 7.34

and digestion have improved. It's amazing how the atmosphere at the dining table can affect the remainder of the day or evening. A few stretches before dinner will satisfy more than your appetite, as well as trimming your midriff (Figure 7.34). Try them instead of a diet pill.

While you're waiting for your meal to arrive, a twist will keep you trim (Figure 7.35). Double Knee Lifts under the tablecloth and Pelvic Floor Pull-Ups help to remind you of how good firm abdominals look and feel. You'll be less tempted to gorge!

Release pent-up feelings of fear, anger, hostility, or nervousness with an Executive Stretch or a Coffee Break Stretch. It helps you relax and let go of the hassles of the day. You don't need alcohol to give you a high. Get your highs from UEs. You'll never have to worry about who's driving home or staying awake!

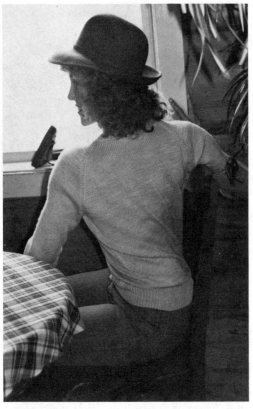

FIGURE 7.35

UNDER THE CLOAK OF ENTERTAINMENT

Watching television can whittle away incredible amounts of your time. Make it a habit to sit on the floor and do your Body Bends and Sitting Twists. They calm you and help you deal with the news. If you have company you can do a few UEs together (Chapter 8).

At the movies you can do your in-line repertoire while waiting to get into the show. Then sit in Tailor Pose or Huggy Pose, or do the Knee-to-Chest Squeeze. Squirm as surreptitiously as you can; don't bother others around you. But to tell you the truth, I'd rather have someone next to me doing a Knee-to-Chest Squeeze than chomping popcorn! The show is a great place to practice your secret Pelvic Floor Pull-Ups coordinated with your breaths.

Watching football, basketball, tennis, and other spectator sports are hard on your back. Carry a back rest with you, or sit correctly in Cosmic Sandwich. Avoid the "spectator slump." If you sit with your elbows rest-

FIGURE 7.36

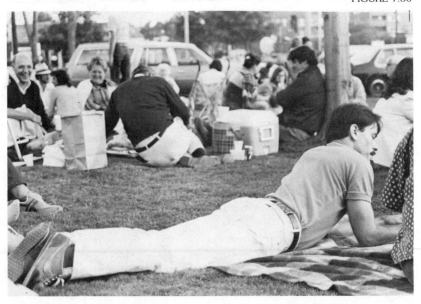

ing on your knees, be careful not to round your back. Make sure your pelvis rotates forward with your spine, as in Seated Forward Bend.

You can do Huggy Pose or twists to help elongate your back and stretch out the kinks. Other good spectator UEs are Knee-to-Chest Squeeze and Single and Double Leg Lifts.

Outdoor summer concerts are wonderful family outings. The man in Figure 7.36 is in Cobra Pose as he relaxes on the grass. Be sure to use Dynamic Duo to protect your back. Place a pad under your abdomen to help tuck your pelvis and elongate your spine.

Undercover Exercise brings you home again. I was sitting in St. John's Chapel in Cambridge, England, for evensong one summer night. I was in Staff Pose thinking how perfect the wooden benches were for this UE, when I suddenly realized that I felt very much at home in this strange place. The thought came to me "If I am at home in my body, then I am at home anywhere."

8

Under Your Covers

And now here is my secret, a very simple secret. It is
only with the heart that one can see rightly; what is
essential is invisible to the eye.
Antoine de Saint Exupéry, *The Little Prince*

Be very still. Listen to the lub-dub of your heart. Ask your doctor to let you hear it with the stethoscope. Your heart has a rhythm, a work phase and a rest phase. Our lives have a work-rest rhythm too. For every intense work period, our bodies and minds need a time of rest. The *quality,* not the quantity, of rest makes a difference in the quality of our lives.

Our vital energy reserves, personal resources, are like a bank account. Dr. Hans Selye describes them this way: "Our reserves of adaptation energy could be compared to an inherited fortune from which we can make withdrawals. . . . We can squander our adaptability recklessly, or we can learn to make this valuable resource last long, by using it wisely and sparingly, only for things that are worthwhile and cause least distress." [9]

We need to be very choosy about how we spend our reserves of vital energy. When we choose to stew over the nit-picky stuff, we're making a withdrawal from that bank account. Our reserves, like those of our

planet—can be depleted. Kenneth R. Pelletier, M.D., in his fascinating book, *Mind as Healer, Mind as Slayer,* gives this advice: "Each person should learn to identify the major stressors in his or her life, to know when stress has reached a dangerous level of duration or intensity, how it is affecting him or her physiologically, and above all, what methods to use to alleviate stress."

You already know some of the most powerful methods for alleviating stress. You've experienced the physical and mental turnaround that UEs give you. A breath and a stretch can take you from jitters to calm. Counting Breaths and other breathing techniques give you a moment of choice so that you can act rather than react! You are no longer a victim of your thoughts and reactions. You are in the driver's seat.

So that should make you some kind of super being? Not at all. Just more fully human and aware of your potential. A lot of work is being done on stress and its relationship to our health. Some people thrive on stress and seek it; others are very sensitive to it and are looking for ways to minimize it in their lives.

The subject of stress is a big stressor in itself. The fact that we can alleviate some of our stressors is a two-edged sword. On one hand, it's quite a revolution to recognize that your thoughts create a lot of your stress . . . and that you *can* choose your thoughts. On the other hand, you're stressed by guilt over not being able always to control your thoughts and alleviate stress. What a conundrum! We end up wishing we didn't know what we know!

Take comfort in the fact that we are very complex creatures. We will never completely know ourselves, and thank goodness for the mystery! Be content to know that you can become a better director-producer of your own show. You get to choose where and when you make the big plays. Be aware that every time you decide on a play, you're making a withdrawal from your vital energy reserves. Choose well and make your moves count!

And don't forget that occasionally blowing off steam can be very healthy for you. Everyone sits up and takes notice! But too many big scenes and you lose the effect, as well as more of your vital energy reserves. Take care of yourself after each expenditure. Rest. Restore your soul and cool your heels.

Even with all our knowledge and good intentions, we sometimes break down and need concentrated healing time. How can you help yourself recuperate?

UNDER THE WEATHER

It was a dark and rainy night. Standing in his driveway, Joel looked up and saw a truck rolling toward him. He jumped out of the way just in time. Joel was lucky and survived the incident with only minor bruises and neck and back pain.

Mary was devastated when she found out she had breast cancer. After the mastec-tomy, she needed daily exercises to get her arms above her head and make her feel attractive and worthwhile again.

At 74, Esther is a healthy and busy lady. But she found herself laid up in bed for three solid weeks with the flu. She needed something to promote healing and keep up her spirits.

We can rant and rage at the down-time, or we can take advantage of it. Recuperating is often the only time-out society permits us to take. We don't often have the courage to "call in well," as Tom Robbins puts it in *Even Cowgirls Get the Blues*. So call in sick and revel in it. Have your friends and family send in chicken soup (better than penicillin) and flowers, massage your feet, and listen to your preoccupation with your injury or ailment. Or you can go into seclusion and take refuge in time by yourself. Some people feel that recuperation is the only way they can get to be by themselves for a while!

Be Sick-Get Better UEs

You and your doctor are partners in healing. Discuss your questions, feelings, and needs with him or her. Decide together on the best course of action for your recovery. Then engage the world's finest physician, your very own body. After pinpointing the areas that need special attention, assist your body's healing power with the three essentials. Increase *circulation; align* your body, mind, and spirit; and create *extension*. The Be Sick-Get Better UEs will do that for you.

One of the first things you'll need to do to get well is to breathe! Get oxygen into your system and move the waste products out. Use your three breathing exercises from Chapter 2. Start with the Observation Breath, then begin Abdominal Breathing, and as soon as you're able, do Rhythmical Complete Breathing.

Then use the slow, continuous movements of the suggested UEs to assist your body's lymphatic system (the "clean-up committee"), autoimmune defense system as well as your body's detoxification system.

In Relaxation Pose or meditation, the body is in its most healing state. Balance and harmony can fill your entire being. When you're in this quiet state, hold in your mind the concept of healing and wellness. Stay with it for 10 to 15 minutes. Repeat the meditation at least three times throughout the day.

The Humming Breath can be used as a healing vibration reaching every cell of your body. Sound vibrations can open you up to healing life-force. Hum on a tone that feels right for you. Think of the vibrations as very strong, capable of breaking through walls of harmful bacteria and infection.

Any of your breathing exercises can be used to direct healing relaxation to tense or injured parts of your body. As you inhale, draw in strength and energy. As you exhale, send that healing power to those healing areas. Inhale hope. Exhale faith. Let your rhythmical breathing calm and center you, allowing your body's amazing power to heal itself.

Norman Cousins used the power and energy of laughter to help himself heal [10]. (Figure 8.1) Laughing oxygenates every cell of your body! Consider the circulation increase. A real treasure is someone who makes you laugh!

Keep your body in alignment so that all of your parts are receiving life-force energy. Align yourself with your spiritual center. As my father observed, "When we're flat on our backs, we are forced to look up." Maybe that's the healing power that gets us on our feet again.

Use this down-time to practice the Counting Breaths, Humming Breath, Gift of Life Breath, Love Missile, and Empathy Observation. They align you with your power source. Also review Relaxation Breaks in Chapter 6. The Love Missile and Empathy Observation can help you resolve the personal conflicts that often make us sick.

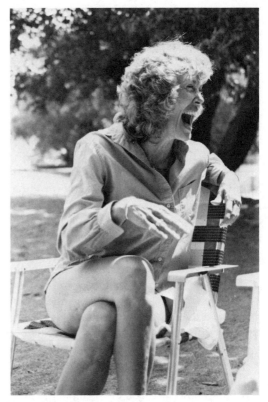

FIGURE 8.1

When you're sick, you want to just curl up and die. You're aching and hurting. UEs will extend you so that the life force can flow through you, soothing and healing you. This extension will help eliminate the blocks in your body that may have caused the illness or inhibits your recovery. Yes, it does take a monumental effort to move when you're sick. As one student said, "If you just get started, you'll feel so much better!"

People report back to us that they thought it was impossible to help themselves heal. One man wrote, "I've got to hand it to you, Mardi. I really didn't believe you, but I tried it. I can't believe how much better I feel. In fact, I feel better than I've ever felt!"

Well, this is it. Here is your Be Sick-Get Better program. Look through the four groups of UEs for ones that you can do. The

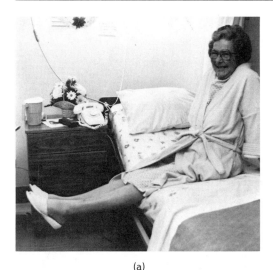

(a)

FIGURE 8.2

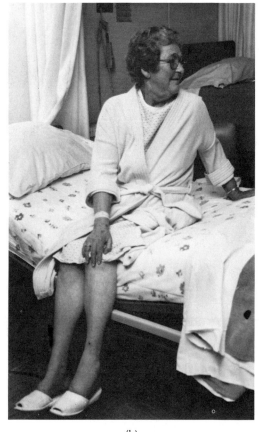

(b)

UEs are grouped so that you can easily refer to those you do while lying on your back, on your stomach, sitting, or when you're up and about. (See Figure 8.2A—B.) Have your doctor help you decide which ones are best for your particular condition. Then slowly and with the utmost awareness, practice one at a time. Remember to pay full attention to how your practice them and give yourself time to extend, stretch, twist, and relax in each UE. All the UEs are described in Chapter 3.

These same Undercover Exercises can bring life and fun to people in nursing homes. Left without stimulation and movement, they become clumsy and listless. Just a simple program of UEs done together in a group can be a shot in the arm for everyone. The greatest benefits, by the way, go to the teacher who works with these sometimes forgotten people. Make up songs and jingles to go with the movements. The rituals for sleep and the partner UEs that follow in this chapter are applicable to the hospital and nursing-home patient. Hats off to all of you who make days brighter and happier for convalescents!

That brings up the question of how to help relatives or friends who are sick or injured. What do you do? What do you say? What should you bring them?

Just take yourself . . . and reach out and touch. Hold a hand or grasp a shoulder if it's appropriate. Be sensitive and respect the person's privacy. You don't have to make a big

Be Sick-Get Better UEs

Supine (on your back)	Prone (on your abdomen)	Sitting	Up and About
*1. Breathing Exercises	1. Cobra Pose	*1. Staff Pose (prop yourself	*1. Mountain Pose
2. Supine Tip and Tuck	(as described in Chapter 2)	against headboard or pillow)	*2. One-Legger
*3. Knee-to-Chest Squeeze	2. Half Bow, Full Bow	2. Knee-to-Chest Squeeze	3. Tree Pose
*4. Huggy Pose	*3. Child's Pose	in Staff Pose	*4. Standing Eagle
*5. Turkey Pose	*4. Cat Stretch	3. Sit Back	5. Mogul
6. Supine One-Legger		(lift feet off bed one at a time)	6. Hot Dog
7. Supine Jackknife		4. Boat Pose	7. 90° Forward Bend
8. Neck Press		(support back with pillows)	8. Dog Stretch
9. Head Roll-Up		5. Bound Angle	9. Triangle
10. Torso Curls		(against headboard or chair)	10. Split-Leg Forward Bend
11. Easy Back Twists		6. Sitting Eagle	*11. One-Step Backbend
12. Supine Torso Twists		7. Eagle Balance	
*13. Relaxation Pose		8. Sitting Twists	
and meditation		9. Roofer's Twist	
		10. Sitting Leg Stretch	
		*11. Relaxation Pose	
		and meditation	

*Easy, beginning UE

deal out of it. Hold a hand or arm and just be with the person. Gently, but firmly, massage the hand or arm. Pretty soon your friend will be relaxed and still. You will be giving the gift of circulation, alignment, and extension. The effects of massage, like UEs, provide the three essentials.

As Barbara K. Koplan, photographer of this book and author of *The Message of Massage,* says: "Trust that as the sea needs no tutoring for her tides to flow, your hands need no credentials to massage. . . . You already know how. The knowledge lies within you and the artist is fully equipped for its expression." [11]

Share some of the UEs with your friend. Better yet, bring a copy of *Undercover Exercise.* Do some UEs together . . . you'll find yourselves laughing together.

It's so easy to get depressed and feel lonely when you're confined to a bed. UEs can stay with your friend from morning to night . . . until your next visit! Here again, I'm drawing on my father's wisdom and experience: "You must accept the patient as he is, not as you might like him to be. And then probe for the resources that can be used in the healing process."

Sometimes illness and injury end in recovery. Other times, the bedside vigil ends in separation. I know the agony and the ecstasy of standing by a loved one valiantly fighting for life. In that struggle you learn to value the little things. I learned to appreciate the gifts of being able to swallow, to move my body, and for that matter, my bowels by myself.

I could never have gotten through those difficult months of my mother's terminal battle without my debriefing, reenergizing workout time. But I didn't know then that I could do UEs during those weary hours at her bedside.

I don't know what we would have done without the doctors, nurses, and true friends who stood by us. Even in her illness, mother's spirit touched us all. The nurses called her

Angel. She taught me, day after day, lessons I had never learned when she was well. Dad's sermons were written at her bedside for nine long months. So were many of his poems that express the pain and hope of human suffering. These three verses are from a longer poem that expresses our experience of the vigil . . . and the final outcome.

GIVING THANKS

Swift weeks of probing and unproven remedies,
a frantic pleasure here and there
then the siren's shrill shriek
the sudden stop
the sudden stop—of a sarcophagus on wheels!

As many days and as many nights?

I cannot tell . . .
but the vigil by her bed will know an end;
then grief anew,
the final ritual,
the solitary track to home,
the facing of northwest winds—alone!

Giving thanks I said? . . .

for a hope that forward looks and
though stripped to quivering flesh
leaves me—even more than yesterday,
a feeling friend
of sorrow's awesome company.

—C.W.A. Bredemeier

Sickness, injury, and death have their places in our lives, their own lessons to teach. They leave us "even more than yesterday, a feeling friend of sorrow's awesome company."

By embracing grief as well as joy, you claim your full range of human experiences. And as we share the inner doubts, grief, and joy with each other, we establish ties that bind us together in love and hope.

RITUALS FOR A PEACEFUL AND SOUND SLEEP

The rest phase of your life deserves the same thought and planning you give the active phase. Remember that it's the quality, not the quantity, of rest that makes a quality life. You know about Sneaky Breaks, Big Breaks, and Relaxation Breaks. Now let's give attention to your longest break, your sleep phase.

Most researchers stress the need for 5 to 8 hours of sleep per night. Anything too much to the plus or minus side of that amount can be potentially unhealthy. Too little sleep wears out the system. Too much sleep means there's an imbalance in the system. Give some thought to this very vital phase of your circadian rhythm. It's your renewal time. Know your own sleep needs. How long do you need to sleep to feel alive, alert, aware, and functioning at your best?

Observing rituals gives a sense of time set apart from all the rest. Give your attention to bedtime rituals that give you the proper rites of passage from an active day into a passive night's sleep. How you awaken often depends on the frame of mind in which you went to sleep.

There are three kinds of rituals described here: Tub, Personal, and Partner. Choose which rituals best fit your lifestyle. To keep a ritual alive, change it; inject it with new life and meaning.

Tub Rituals

The old-fashioned bathtub can be a spa in your own home and on the road. Nothing can be so comforting as a warm bath. It's too good to be forgotten. Your tub ritual can soak out the problems of your day, melting away tension and stress. It's an ideal place to create more length in your hamstrings and strength in your abdominals.

Prepare your bath with style! You can turn down the lights and use your favorite suds, scents, mineral salts, or baking soda. Now enjoy!

Sitting Forward Bend   Use the warmth of the water to help your rotate your pelvis forward. Bend your knees and bring your ribs to your thighs. Gradually straighten your legs and see if you can keep your ribs in contact with your thighs (Figure 8.3). Feel your pelvis rotating into a tipped position. Hold onto a washcloth looped around your feet to help you stretch. Breathe into your stretch and relax. This is one time you can really enjoy a forward bend.

Knee-to-Chest Squeeze   Lean back against the tub and draw one knee at a time to your

FIGURE 8.3

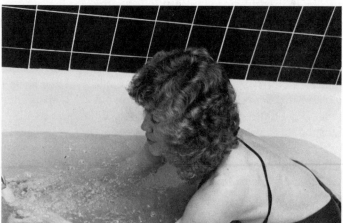

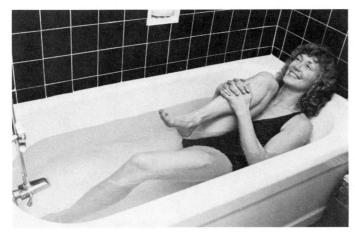

FIGURE 8.4

chest (Figure 8.4), breathing rhythmically with the squeeze-release.

Sitting Twist Follow the directions for these two stretches in Configuration 6. You can use the sides of the tub to push-pull against (Figure 8.5).

Sit Back or Boat Sit in Staff Pose and then lean against the back of the tub. Bring your knees to your chest and lift your feet one at a time off the floor of the tub. Apply Cosmic Sandwich. Press your elbows against the sides or back of the tub and straighten one or both legs for Boat.

Tip and Tuck Lean back against the tub. Lift and lower folded arms or keep both arms straight as you tip and tuck your pelvis. Notice the relationship between contracting and relaxing muscles as you tip and tuck for several breaths. The warm tub is a wonderful place to do this.

Neck Press Slide down into the water until you're up to your neck in hot water! Then press the back of your neck against the tub. Tip and tuck your chin with your breathing.

Cobra Pose Turn over on your abdomen and work in Dynamic Duo. Stretch your arms

upward and press against the wall or tub (Figure 8.6). Bend your knees if the tub isn't long enough to keep them straight. The water will help you do a good pelvic tuck using abdominals and pelvic floor muscles.

These are just a few of the possibilities for tub UEs. Again, you're limited only by your inventiveness. Make it up as you go!

Relaxation Roll over onto your back again and breathe rhythmically. Rest quietly. You will sleep like an angel tonight!

When you're soaking in hot water, be

FIGURE 8.5

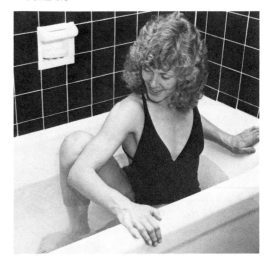

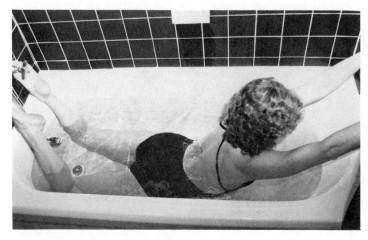

FIGURE 8.6

aware of dehydration. Don't stay in the tub if you feel faint or overheated. Replace lost fluids and electrolytes with diluted juices.

If you have a hot tub, use it to soak up your troubles. Do One-Legger Stretches, Bound Angle, and Eagle Balance. Work with a partner on the UEs described later on in this chapter, like Triangle, Warrior, and Sitting Eagle Rock. Refer to Chapter 5 for workout routines in water.

Personal Rituals: A Way to Relieve Insomnia

Take time to unwind before you go to sleep. Be with yourself, by yourself. Your Tub Ritual may be a way to do that. Here are some other ways.

What you do and think, particularly in the last two hours before sleep, influences the quality of your sleep. Don't watch frightening movies or upsetting news and expect to have a good night's sleep. I think that one of the reasons Johnny Carson and "Mash" have lasted so long is that they make people laugh. They help you forget the heavies of your own problems.

If you're having trouble getting to sleep or are waking during the night, look at what you are eating, drinking, doing, and thinking about. Go over your last waking hours before you go to bed. Are they peaceful or trauma-

tic? If you like to watch the evening news, see if it's affecting your sleep adversely. If so, you could watch the news earlier in the day or read the paper tomorrow. You can also do your bedtime UEs while watching the news or your favorite program. They help you stay warmly detached, calm and centered. We all make a significant contribution to world affairs by being involved and caring, but bedtime is not the time to get all agitated! You'll end up stewing all night. If you spend a sleepless night tonight, you can't act effectively tomorrow.

Read and Reflect   Choose enlightening and uplifting literature. The faith and struggles of others inspire us. Feel a part of that company of pilgrims and pioneers who have persisted in the past and those who persist now.

Meditate   Spend some quiet time being still and listening to your inner voice. If you go to sleep at night with someone else's ideas hammering in your brain and you wake to yet another's on the radio, how will you ever hear your own voice?

Use the meditative guides in Chapter 2. Spend 15 to 20 minutes in quiet stillness. Review your day briefly. A great day? Be grateful! Or perhaps it wasn't your best. Reflect on why and what you can do next time to change it. Take note of the risks you took and how you fared. Then be still and listen to your inner teacher.

Bedtime UEs Now crawl into bed and do these Undercover Exercises for 7 minutes. Add a 5- to 15-minute Relaxation Pose and you have a 12- to 22-minute investment in a good night's sleep.

1. Supine Tip and Tuck
2. Knee-to-Chest Squeeze
3. Supine One-Legger
4. Jackknife
5. Supine Eagle
6. Easy Back Twists
7. Fetal Pose
8. Relaxation Pose

Go to sleep with the knowledge that the same consciousness and energy that guides you through the day will guide you through the night. It never slumbers and will be very close to you when you awaken, even closer than your breath.

MAKING LOVE LOVELY

If you think this is all about sex under the covers, you're right. If you think it's another how-to manual, you're wrong.

Making love lovely is about discovering (1) how much we really like each other; (2) the joy and headaches we share; and (3) the strength and encouragement we give each other to be our best selves.

Here are ways to explore all the dimensions of ourselves with each other. Couples can use them to enrich their love-making. Families can use them to increase their level of communication. And business associates can use them to "conspire with and for each other." [12] They establish ties that bind us together, not out of greed, but in love and service to each other (Figure 8.7).

The "me first" binge of the past two decades has left us sick of looking out for number one. Something in our heart of hearts tells us that, like our forefathers, we'd better hang together or surely we'll hang separately.

What is essential to making love lovely is invisible to the eye. In *The Little Prince*, the fox tells the Little Prince that to make friends, or tame, means to establish ties: "If you tame me, then we shall need each other. To me, you will be unique in all the world. To you, I shall be unique in all the world. . . ." [13]

How do you approach making love lovely? With celebration! Make it a ritual that sets this time aside from any other time. This is a time exclusively for you, as couples, friends, families, teams. Everything else is put on hold, tabled during this time. Even if it's for only a few moments, quality time is better than quantity.

Establish ties. Discover the uniqueness of what you offer each other. Consistently and persistently allow each other room to grow and change. The secret? It is seeing with the heart. With warmth and encouragement allow each the right to make mistakes and learn from them. It takes miles and miles and miles of heart to allow each person the time

FIGURE 8.7

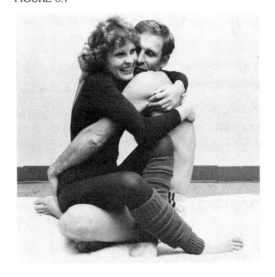

and space to experience the cause and effect of his or her behavior. It's much easier to interfere and try to change the inevitable outcome. Real love means that we stand by and support, but not prevent, the growth of those we love.

Reach out and hold each other, touch each other. Without touch, we all die. Let Barbara K. Koplan's message encourage you to massage those tired shoulders, arms, hands, or feet. As she says, you already know how to massage. A neck and shoulder massage can be better than roses on your birthday. Well, almost! After a hard day of gardening or working in the yard, give each other a back massage. Or how about the pièce de resistance—a foot massage! Just remember the three essentials and visualize your hands increasing blood flow to the area, aligning the body parts, and extending the muscles for proper energy flow. Give each other the gift of touch.

Breathing Together
Sit back to back for the next three breathing UEs.

Simple Breathing Awareness Sit in Tailor Pose, your ankles crossed, with your backs and heads touching. If your hips don't touch, sit on cushions, as in Staff Pose (Chapter 3). Breathe several rhythmical breaths together. As you inhale, feel your back ribs pressing toward the back of your partner. As you exhale, feel your ribs coming away from your partner's back.

Cat-Cow Breathing In the same position, loosely clasp fingers or index fingers. If your shoulders are too stiff, grasp a tie or belt in each hand, and then hold on to your partner's tie. Lift your arms as you do in Supine Tip and Tuck, but this time lift them together (Figure 8.8). Inhale as you lift, Cow Pose. Exhale as you lower, Cat Pose. After several cycles of breathing together, release hands and sit with your backs still touching. Experience the energy and warmth of each other.

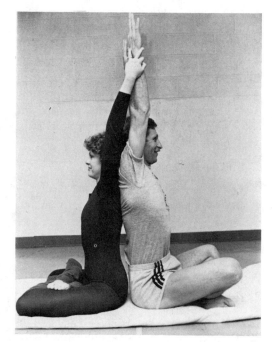

FIGURE 8.8

Rocking Chair Link arms together at the elbows. *Gently* and *slowly* rock backward and forward (Figure 8.9). Feel the rhythmical movements of your bodies. The person rocking forward exhales and tips the pelvis forward. The person rocking backward inhales and tucks the pelvis backward. Rock together for a few moments. Then sit still and enjoy the effects of rocking.

Now turn around and sit face to face for the next three breathing UEs.

Contemplating Your Navel Sit face to face in Tailor Pose. Stare at each other's navel! Inhale together and exhale together. Watch abdomens swell and recede like waves. Some people will make big waves.

Give and Take Continue as above, sitting in Tailor Pose, except that as one of you inhales, the other exhales. It's like a see-saw. Once you've established a nice rhythm, feel the give and take that symbolizes how you give and

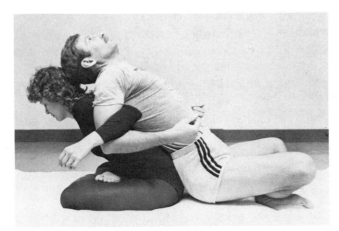

FIGURE 8.9

take with each other. Then, holding hands or arms, gently rock backward and forward. Exhale forward as your partner inhales backward. Feel the exchange of energy as you inhale and exhale.

Sitting Eagle Rock Separate your legs as for Sitting Eagle. The person with the shorter legs or tighter hamstrings will need to place the feet to the inside of the partner's legs. Then one of you rocks forward, tipping your pelvis, while the other rocks backward, tucking the pelvis (Figure 8.10). Tip for forward bending, tuck for backward bending. Breathe and rock together, as in Give and Take, receiving your partner's breath and then giving it back again.

UEs Together

Any partnership is a soul-stretching adventure, with emphasis on "stretching." Working together for a common good is a mission that

FIGURE 8.10

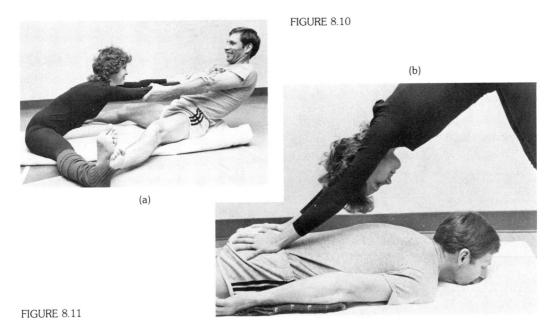

(a)

(b)

FIGURE 8.11

stretches our horizons. We need each other to complement our inadequacies, for feedback on how we're doing, and to reassure and support each other.

Doing UEs together doubles the fun and benefits. Words are often a source of misunderstanding, but UEs together can help us to understand each other in new ways. They help us to open and share in ways that have been difficult or painful. Sometimes the communication is beyond words and nothing needs to be said. Child to parent, parent to child, friend to friend, lover to lover . . . UEs together are a rich investment.

One of you is *A* and the other *B* in the UEs together.

Bound Angle

- Sit back to back. *A* sits in Bound Angle, *B* in Tailor Pose.
- *B* places the hands on *A*'s thighs; near the groin if *A*'s groin is tight, near the knees if *A*'s groin can take a lot of stretch.
- Inhale together. As you exhale, *B* presses gently downward on *A*'s thighs.
- Keep backs together in Cosmic Sandwich. Breathe and stretch together.
- Now *A* moves forward into a forward bend. *B* helps *A* by pressing downward on *A*'s thighs and leaning against *A*'s back.
- Sometimes *B* has to bring knees together and press soles of feet to the floor. *B* may lift the hips off the floor.
- Change positions and repeat.

Dog Stretch

- *A* and *B* take Table Pose with hands interlaced and crowns of heads touching.
- Inhale together.
- Exhaling together, lift hips and straighten legs. Keep heads touching.

- Inhale together.
- Exhaling, stretch hips and heads away from each other. Push away from your interlaced hands.
- Hold and work the Dog Stretch, feeling each other's energy.
- Take time to stretch away from each other, always mindful of the support and energy you receive and give in your relationship.
- Exhale down into Table Pose and then Cat Stretch.
- Does this UE remind you of how often you butt heads?!

Cobra Pose

- *A* lies on the floor in Cobra Pose. Place a cushion under your hips as described in Chapter 3.
- *A* exhales and elongates the spine. *B* watches *A* and checks *A*'s body position. Is the spine elongated? Is Dynamic Duo in effect?
- *B* stands at the head of *A* and places the hands on *A*'s pelvis.
- *B* goes into Dog Stretch, hands pressing on *A*'s pelvis helping it to rotate backward. (See Figure 8.11.)
- Then *B* returns to a squate and grasps *A*"s wrists, pulling *A*'s arms out beyond *A*'s head.
- On an exhalation, *B* *gently* and *slowly* stretches *A*'s arms upward and away from *A*'s pelvis, elongating the back.
- On an exhalation, *B* *gently* and *slowly* stretches *A*'s arms upward and away from *A*'s pelvis, elongating the back.
- Return arms to the floor; change places and repeat.
- You can also use a broom handle instead of holding onto wrists. *B* holds the handle between *A*'s hands and then gently and slowly pulls the handle outward.

- This is a wonderful stretch for the ribs and a great test of your application of Dynamic Duo.

The Gate

- Kneel together side by side. Leave a little space between you.
- Stretch your outer leg to the side as you would for Triangle. Point toes or rest your heels on the floor.
- Observe all the alignment principles you learned in Back and Body Trainers.
- Clasp your inside hands together.
- Inhale and lift your inside arms overhead.
- Exhale and apply Cosmic Sandwich.
- Inhale and raise your outer arms to shoulder level.
- As in Triangle, exhale and push your hips to the side, this time toward each other. Your hips may or may not touch.
- Exhaling, go into Triangle in opposite directions. Your inner arms and torso form a diamond. You're still holding hands.
- Drop the outer arm and rest the hand on your lower leg. See Figure 8.12.
- Hold and breathe.
- Exhale up and change sides.
- This UE reminds me of a Pueblo Indian wedding vase. There is a union at the base while the two vessels branch out to form two separate parts . . . still united at the base.

Intense Forward Bend

- Stand in Mountain Pose back to back with feet several inches apart. Adjust the distance to your needs.
- Exhale and bow away from each other in a 90° Forward Bend.
- Hold there and elongate your spine. You can bend knees, but don't round your lower back.

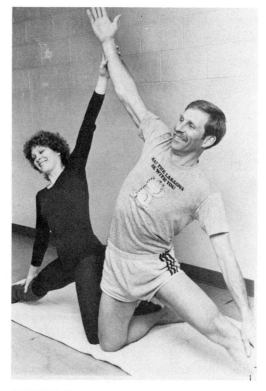

FIGURE 8.12

- Then stretch out and downward toward the floor.
- Reach back and grasp each others hands or arms. Keep your spines elongated. Bend your knees if you need to, and maintain cosmic Sandwich.
- When you can stretch farther, reach for each other's shins or ankles. See Figure 8.13.
- Breathe there, letting the warmth of your partner's legs help lengthen your stubborn hamstrings.
- Exhale back to 90° Forward Bend and then back to Mountain Pose.

Tree Pose

- Stand side by side in Mountain Pose. Maintain 6 to 12 inches distance between you.

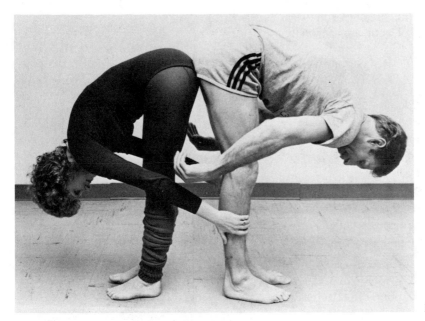

FIGURE 8.13

- Stand on inside legs and clasp inside hands.
- Move into Tree Pose together. Lift your outer foot and press it against your inner thigh. Reach down with your free hand and assist your foot onto the thigh.
- Balance together. Laughing helps!
- Inhaling, lift your inside arms with hands clasped.
- Exhaling, place your outer hands together in front of you, forming the Namaste hand position. (You may want to look back at Figure 6.35, p. 138.)
- Namaste. Greet with respect the oneness of two.
- Breathe together. Notice how your roots support each other, how you can branch out and up but still be firm at your roots.
- Exhaling, come out of Tree Pose.
- Change sides and repeat.

Warrior

- Stand back to back in Mountain Pose.
- Step forward with your right legs.

- Move your left leg back behind your partner's right heel.
- Inhale and clasp hands.
- Exhale into Lunge position, knees forming right angles.
- Tuck your pelvis.
- Inhale and lift arms together.
- Exhale and create Dynamic Duo.
- Feel your strength as you stretch back to back as warriors (Figure 8.14). Together you can face anything!
- Exhale and come out of Warrior by straightening your legs and dropping arms.
- Repeat on the other side.

Supine One-Legger

- *A* lies on the floor in alignment. Exhaling, lift one leg for a hamstring stretch. The leg remaining on the floor, base leg, can be bent or straight.
- *Very carefully* and *gently*, B encourages A's leg to extend even farther. Slowly and with awareness, guide A's raised

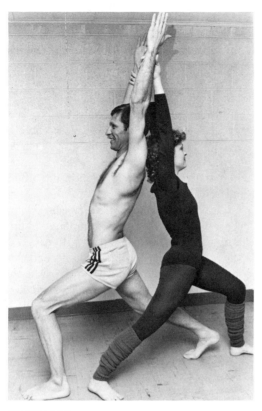

FIGURE 8.14

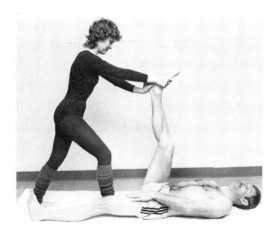

FIGURE 8.15

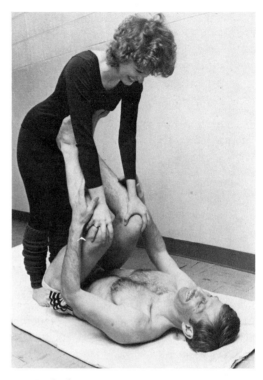

FIGURE 8.16

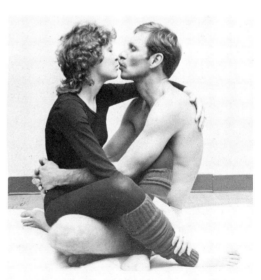

FIGURE 8.17

leg, either bent or straight, toward the head (Figure 8.15). This gentle pressure will help the hamstrings stretch even further.

- Switch legs and repeat.
- Switch positions and A helps B.

Huggy Pose

- A does Huggy Pose.
- B places hands on A's feet or legs and gently leans on A's legs to help flatten and lengthen the back. Don't flop on A but gently press against the legs (Figure 8.16).
- B can gradually increase pressure as A relaxes into the stretch.

Making love lovely brings new dimensions to being together. Enjoy being together, learning from each other, and appreciating yourselves in new ways. Henry and Terry, pictured in these partner UEs, have been working together like this for two years. Terry has changed her swayback posture and made major changes in her life. Henry has loosened stiff shoulders, straightened his back, and learned new ways to deal with stress.

When we open ourselves to life, give and receive, and empathize, we are able to enjoy the fullness of human bliss for which we yearn. Any easy substitute leaves us empty and bitter . . . with our relationship abandoned in the corner.

Love is a transforming power (Figure 8.17). It makes the most mundane circumstances sparkle. It means having to say "I'm sorry" and having to graciously accept "I'm sorry." When we love, we are more alive and the realest real we can be. Our lives are filled with the enchantment of a secret hidden in the depths of our being. As the Little Prince knows, "What is essential is invisible to the eye."

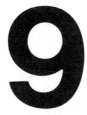

Agents of Influence

Life is no "brief candle" to me. It is a sort of splendid
torch which we have got hold of for the moment, and
we want to make it burn as brightly as possible before
handing it on to future generations.
George Bernard Shaw, "Man and Superman"

YOUR SECRET CODE

You practice it daily in your Winning-Edge
Workout. You feel the warmth and power of it
as you do Double Leg Lifts in your office
chair. You experience its strong, sustaining
support as you do Pelvic Floor Pull-ups just
before you walk to the podium.

Your secret code is the essential that's
invisible to the eye. Like a torch, it burns
within you. Its effects can be seen, felt, and
heard, but the secret code remains a buried
treasure at the foundation of your house. It is
the power of your spiritual center symbolized
by the power of your core body muscles. It
gives you grace and length, agility and beauty
in your movements. *Your secret code is Core
Power—the experience of the infinite at the
core of fitness.*

DECIPHERING YOURSELF

Who am I? This is the age-old question we
have asked ourselves since we first became
aware that we were separate from our moth-
ers. That's where the fear, loneliness, and
alienation began. As we grow, we have to
walk the difficult way back to oneness, to
being with each other in ways that recognize
our individual, as well as collective, identity.

We can learn about ourselves in relationships. We hold up a mirror for each other
(Figure 9.1). Together we find ourselves and
give each other the courage and support to go
on learning.

We also learn who we are by paying
attention to what the body tells us. It can give
us an honest appraisal of the way we were . . .
and are. As you look at your stance in a mirror, you can see very interesting reasons for
your habitual posture, reasons that are deeply
rooted in your personality. Trying to change
your posture without understanding or getting
to the cause is usually a waste of time. It's the
chicken and egg riddle again. Is your attitude
changing your posture, or is your posture
changing your attitude? Your Winning-Edge
Workout is helping you practice new ways of
standing, sitting, and moving. *UEs give you*

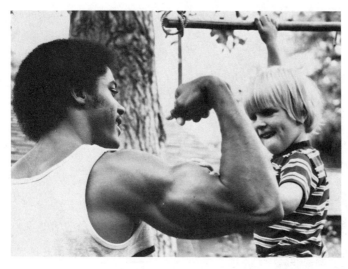

FIGURE 9.1

powerful new ways to exorcise old stuff. They give you options for change.

BREAKING THE CODE OF CONVENTION

How is it possible that we will fight for our personal freedom, campaign against injustice, strike for benefits . . . and still live in the prisons of our own bodies?

Undercover Exercise breaks the code of conventional rigidity, dis-ease, and apathy. It is a revolution against the chains and bars that confine and restrict us in our own houses. All it takes is a glimmer of light, a breakthrough in some rigidity, and we know what we've been missing.

The training ground of the Undercover Agent is the check and balance system. In the Winning-Edge Workout, the intelligence of the body teaches you the dangers of excess. You know about it when you go overboard . . . pain and discomfort! The rigors of daily discipline save us from the fanaticism of excess.

Consciously or unconsciously we make our choices to do things the same old way or break old habits by trying something different.

We can succumb to gravity and let it pull us down, or use it to grow up. We can live life as victims, or have a mission that turns everydayism into adventure. (Figure 9.2 and Figure 3.113, p. 81.)

FIGURE 9.2

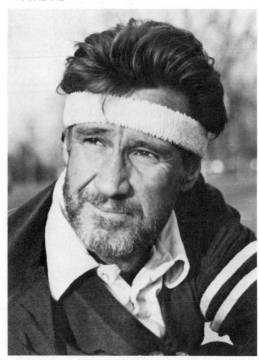

This is the code that breaks the grip of conventionality and sums up *Undercover Exercise*.

1. Tip and Tuck with every task, walk in Cosmic Sandwich, reach in Dynamic Duo.
2. Stay flexible. Do UEs to change direction or to give you the endurance to keep your course.
3. The world is your playground. Work out wherever you are and with whatever you've got.
4. Sitting? Keep your knees a little higher than your hips. Squirm!
5. Standing? Put one foot up every chance you get, and don't stand still.
6. Keep your body in alignment.
7. Let your breath move you.
8. Be still in the silence of your center . . . even though you may be surrounded by noise and confusion.
9. Do the best that you can with the best that you have to be the best that you are!
10. Stay in the net!

"Stay in the net." Stay in radio contact with your home base, colleagues, and fellow agents. Your success and survival depend on staying in touch with those who, like you, are seeking quality and excellence in their lives.

A log that falls away from the fire doesn't burn very long. When you are isolated and out of contact, you lose your spark. Keep track of each other. Be interested, concerned, and supportive. Use the three essentials to keep your relationships, as well as your body, healthy.

Circulation. Get around. Know what's going on. Current thoughts, struggles, and the campaigns of others can be vitally important to your mission.

Alignment. Align yourself with people of excellence in all walks of life. Pace them. Be one with them. Practice empathy.

Extension. Reach out and extend yourself. Be a real friend. Even when it's tough, be there.

The confidential files of other agents of influence reveal their struggles, their accomplishments, their missions.

Leon Jaworski. "That taught me to cross the barrier of doing things that were unpopular, to live with them and to realize that after the ordeal is over, you feel inner satisfaction that you have done your duty. [14]"

Mary Mulligan. "When I feel as if I can't make the wheels go 'round one more time, I remember to breathe deeply into my legs. Somehow new strength flows into me and I know I can make it."

George Bernard Shaw. "This is the true joy in life . . . the being a force of nature instead of a feverish selfish little clod of ailments and grievances complaining that the world will not devote itself to making you happy. [15]"

C.W.A. Bredemeier. "I dare to dream of peace—midst deepening gloom, / the nations piling up for overkill, in nuclear holocaust to hasten doom . . . Ah, let me dream, and pray, and work . . . until! [16]"

Agents of influence, what a mighty and awsome company! Our paths may be diverse, divergent, and difficult. But with our talent and wit, experience and determination, we can make a difference in whether we and this planet survive.

All Points Bulletin to All Undercover Agents

"It's not the wind; it's the way you set your sail."

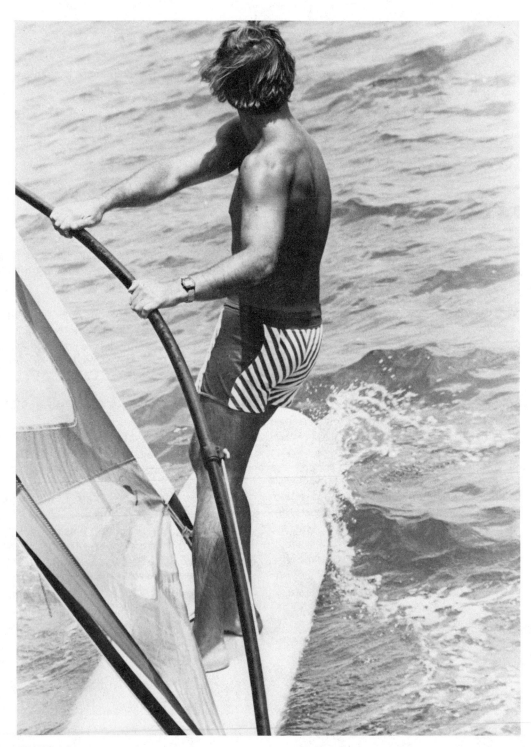

FIGURE 9.3

Bibliography

Anthony, Catherine Parker, and Norma Jane Kolthoff, *Textbook of Anatomy and Physiology,* 8th Ed., St. Louis: The C. V. Mosby Company, 1971.

Bredemeier, C.W.A., "I Dare to Dream of Peace," unpublished poem, 1982. [16]

Bredemeier, C.W.A., "Giving Thanks," unpublished poem, 1969.

Cailliet, Rene, *Low Back Pain Syndrome,* 3rd Ed., Philadelphia: F. A. Davis Company, 1981.

Cooper, Kenneth, H., *The Aerobics Program for Total Well Being,* New York: M. Evans and Co., 1982.

Cousins, Norman, *Human Options,* New York: Norton, 1981. (Also published as *Healing & Belief,* Mosaic Press, 1982.)

Cousins, Norman, *Anatomy of an Illness as Seen Through the Eyes of the Patient,* New York: Bantam Books, 1981. [10]

Daniels, Lucille, and Catherine Worthingham, *Therapeutic Exercise for Body Align-ment and Function,* 2nd ed., Philadelphia: W. B. Saunders Company, 1977.

de Saint Exupèry, Antoine, *The Little Prince,* New York: Harcourt Brace and World Inc. 1943. [13]

Ferguson, Marilyn, *The Aquarian Conspiracy: Personal and Social Transformation in the 1980's,* Los Angeles: J. P. Tarcher, Inc., 1980. [12, p. 417]

Gardner, John, *Excellence: Can We Be Equal and Excellent Too?* New York: Harper and Row, 1971.

Iyengar, B.K.S., *Light on Yoga,* Rev. ed., New York: Schocken Books, 1979.

Iyengar, B.K.S., *Light on Pranayama,* New York: The Crossroads Publishing Company, 1981. [4, p. 20].

Jaworsky, Leon, *Rocky Mountain News,* 10 Dec. 1982. [14, p. 3]

Kapandji, I.A., *The Physiology of the Joints,* New York: Churchill Livingston, Longman Inc., 1974, reprinted 1979.

Kapit, Wynn and Lawrence M. Elson, *The Anatomy Coloring Book, New York: Harper and Row, 1977.*

Keller, Helen, *The Story of my Life,* New York: Doubleday, 1954.

Koplan, Barbara K., *The Message of Massage,* Denver: Humanics Co., 1982. [11]

Kraus, Hans, *The Cause, Prevention and Treatment of Backache, Stress and Tension,* New York: Simon and Schuster, Inc., 1965. (Pocket Books, 1969, 1976.)

Krishnamurti, J., *Krishnamurti's Journal,* New York: Harper and Row, 1982.

Lewis, C.S., "Inklings" (letter to Arthur Greeves), Dobbs Ferry, New York: Cahill and Company, 1982. [8]

Lindbergh, Anne Morrow, *A Gift From the Sea,* New York: Random House, 1978.

Luby, Sue, *Hatha Yoga for Total Health,* Englewood Cliffs, NJ: Prentice-Hall, Inc., 1978.

Merton, Thomas, "Extemporaneous Remarks," *The World Religions Speak On,* in Raymond Bailey, *Thomas Merton on Mysticism,* Garden City, New York: Image Books, 1975.

Merton, Thomas, *New Seeds of Contemplation,* New York: New Directions Publishing Corporation, 1972. [5, p. 3]

Naisbitts, John, "John Naisbitts Monitors a Changing America," *The Tarrytown Letter,* Tarrytown, N.Y. (April, 1982), p. 10.

"Nightline," Dr. Stephen Levin, Dr. Bernard Jacobs, "Back Pain," New York: American Broadcasting Companies, Inc., 1982. [1]

Pelletier, Kenneth, *Mind as Healer, Mind as Slayer,* New York: Delacorte, 1977.

Restak, Richard M., *The Self Seekers,* Garden City, New York: Doubleday & Co., Inc., 1982.

Selye, Hans, *Stress Without Distress,* New York: Harper and Row, 1974. [9]

Shaw, George Bernard, *Man and Superman,* New York: Viking Penguin, 1980. [15]

Simmonton, Carl, *Cancer Self-Help Education,* Cancer Counseling and Research Center, Saratoga, CA: Health Education Programs, 1977.

Stewart, Mary, *The Crystal Cave,* New York: Fawcett, 1979.

Taber's Cyclopedic Medical Dictionary, 13th ed., Philadelphia: F. A. Davis Company, 1977.

Tennyson, Alfred Lord, *The Poetic and Dramatic Work of Alfred Lord Tennyson,* Boston: Houghton Mifflin Company, 1898. [3, p. 498]

Tillich, Paul, "Existential Analyses and Religious Symbols," *Classical and Contemporary Readings in the Philosophy of Religion,* 2nd ed., John Hick, ed., Englewood Cliffs, NJ: Prentice-Hall, Inc., 1970. [2, pp. 321-32; 6]

Tolstoy, Leo, *Tolstoy: What Men Live By* New York: Peter Pauper Press, 1954.

Webster's New Collegiate Dictionary, Springfield, Mass: Merriam Company, 1981.

Wells, Katherine F., *Kinesiology: The Scientific Basis of Human Motion,* 4th ed., Philadelphia: W. B. Saunders Company, 1966.

Williams, Paul C., *Low Back and Neck Pain: Causes and Conservation Treatments,* Springfield, Illinois: Charles C. Thomas Publishers, 1974. [7]

White, Ganga, and Anna Forrest, *Double Yoga: A New System for Total Body Health,* New York: Penguin Books, 1981.

Index of
Undercover Exercises

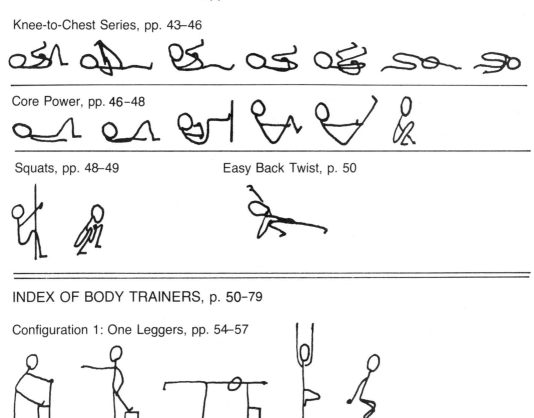
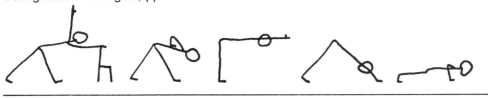
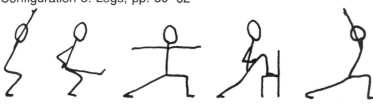

Configuration 4: Body Bends, pp. 62–65

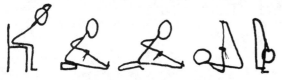

Configuration 5: Spread Eagle, pp. 65–67

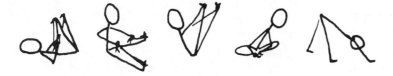

Configuration 6: Torso Twists, pp. 67–69

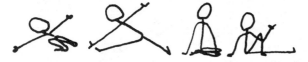

Configuration 7: Bow, pp. 70–73

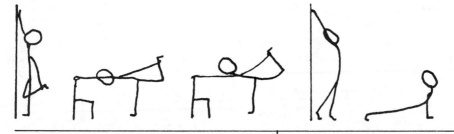

Configuration 8: Bottoms Up, pp. 73–76   Configuration 9: Bar Hangs, pp. 76–77

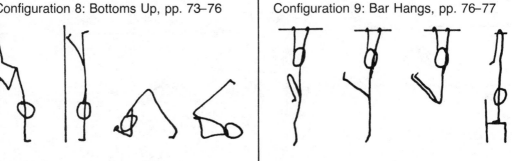

Configuration 10: Sun Power, pp. 77–82,   Sun Swings, pp. 77–79

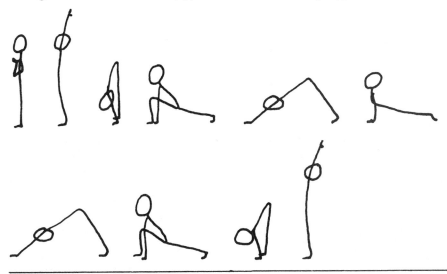

Configuration 10: Sun Power, pp. 77, 82   Jumping Sun, pp. 79–80

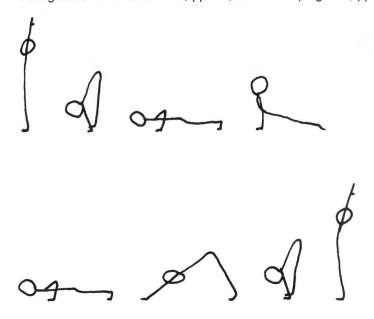

Subject Index